SELF-REGULATION IN EARLY CHILDHOOD

SELF-REGULATION IN EARLY CHILDHOOD

Nature and Nurture

Martha B. Bronson

THE GUILFORD PRESS
New York   London

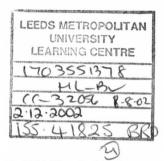
© 2000 The Guilford Press
A Division of Guilford Publications, Inc.
72 Spring Street, New York, NY 10012
www.guilford.com

Printed in the United States of America

This book is printed on acid-free paper.

Last digit is print number: 9 8 7 6 5 4 3 2 1

Library of Congress Cataloging-in-Publication Data

Bronson, Martha.
  Self-regulation in early childhood: nature and nurture / Martha B.
  Bronson.
    p. cm.
  Includes bibliographical references and index.
  ISBN 1-57230-532-0
  1. Self-control in children. 2. Child rearing.   I. Title.
  BF723.S25 B76 2000
  155.4′1825—dc21   99-057183

About the Author

Martha B. Bronson, EdD, is an associate professor of developmental and educational psychology at Boston College, where she directs the early childhood program. She received her bachelor's degree in psychology from Boston University and her master's and doctoral degrees in human development from Harvard University. She has extensive experience in educational evaluation in early childhood, and her observational measures of young children's self-regulatory skills have been used in a number of national studies. Her research focuses on the development of planning and organizing strategies in both social and cognitive mastery situations, and the influence of the environment on the development of these skills. She has also been a teacher of young children and has written *The Right Stuff for Children Birth to 8: Selecting Play Materials to Support Development.*

Contents

Introduction and Overview

The capacity for conscious and voluntary self-regulation is central to our understanding of what it is to be human. It underlies our assumptions about choice, decision making, and planning. Our conceptions of freedom and responsibility depend on it. Among all living things, we hold only ourselves legally and morally accountable for our actions. A tree that falls on our house, insects that destroy our crops, or a dog that bites our child is not considered "responsible" in the same way, though each is capable of some forms of self-regulation. Many of the world's ethical systems suggest that we are also somewhat accountable for our thoughts—that we must not even *wish* evil on others and should "love" our neighbors as well as refrain from actively harming them.

Self-regulation begins with life itself. All living things have self-regulating and self-organizing mechanisms that guide their development and adaptation. They are equipped with a variety of regulatory systems, which help them maintain the biological conditions necessary to sustain life. Animals, especially those higher on the phylogenetic scale, have complex nervous systems. These provide a mix of innately organized regulatory mechanisms and those that can be developed through experience for additional flexibility.

Some animals, such as house flies and jellyfish, must be ready to cope with the environment without help from the time they emerge into the world. They are equipped with a variety of built-in regula-

1

tory functions that, although comparatively "hard-wired" and inflexible, work most of the time. Other creatures, such as rats, dolphins, chimpanzees, and humans, have more educable regulatory systems that can learn to cope with a wider array of environmental circumstances. We pay for this flexibility with an increased need for external support and protection early in life and a need for additional time to learn to survive and adapt.

The human capacity to develop its own self-regulatory systems is impressive. Although the newborn infant is relatively helpless, the potential for developing adaptive control is present from the beginning. Early self-regulation is primarily reactive, with external events and internal biological requirements and reflexes setting the stage for organizing, modifying, and regulating responses. With maturation and experience the child becomes increasingly capable of proactive, planful, and conscious (metacognitive) control. "Experience" includes support and guidance from other people and from the mental and material tool kit provided by culture. Gradually, with this assistance, the child gains control over sensory–motor, emotional, and cognitive systems. She* is increasingly able to direct external behavior and internal thought processes and to successfully influence the social and physical environment.

Significant progress toward self-regulation is made during early childhood. Flavell (1977) describes this progress as "one of the really central and significant cognitive-developmental hallmarks of the early childhood period" (p. 64). During these years the child makes tremendous leaps forward in regulating arousal (Brazelton, 1978; Piaget, 1952) and emotional responses (Eisenberg et al., 1995; Fox, 1994), gaining adaptive control of behavior in familiar settings (Luria, 1961; Mischel & Mischel, 1983; Vygotsky, 1962), and learning to control mental processing and problem solving (Harris, 1990; Vygotsky, 1962; Zivin, 1979). Motivational patterns, which influence both the direction and strength of the child's self-regulatory efforts, are also developed during this period (Deci & Ryan, 1987; Dweck, 1986; Harter, 1981). Underlying this progress are millions of

---

*To avoid repeating the cumbersome construction "he or she" throughout the text, I will use the feminine pronoun. The reader should understand that I am referring to both male and female children, however.

neural networks that support higher-level functioning, which are being formed and pruned in the child's brain during this period of maximum plasticity (Shore, 1997).

This book addresses four major issues in relation to self-regulation in young children: *definition, development, integration,* and *support.* Because early childhood is a period when self-regulation is developing rapidly, in ways that form a basis for later development, it is important to understand what self-regulation is and how to support it. Unfortunately, there is not a single or simple *definition* of this concept, even in relation to young children's everyday functioning in home and school environments. Psychologists often use different words to refer to it (impulse control, self-control, self-management, self-direction, independence, etc.) and describe its development in quite different ways.

Some definitions focus primarily on the control of external behaviors, such as the ability to comply with adult requests or to control behavior and emotions adaptively in particular situations. Many parents and teachers have adopted this view of self-regulation because the control of behavior and emotions is important in both home and school settings. Children who cannot conform to age-appropriate expectations for self-control cause difficulties and generate concern. Descriptions of these kinds of self-regulatory functions are prominent in psychoanalytic theory, behavioral theory, and social learning theory, but the accounts provided do not always agree and the terms used in each theoretical tradition are somewhat different.

Other definitions of self-regulation focus more on the control of cognitive systems, such as the ability to control attention, to direct and monitor thinking and problem solving, and to engage in independent learning activities. Although not always obvious at the youngest ages, the development of cognitive self-regulation begins very early and becomes increasingly important as the child grows older and is expected to take responsibility for her own learning. Developmental psychologists and information-processing theorists have provided a variety of accounts of the development of cognitive control systems.

The characteristics of self-regulation also vary with *age and development.* A child with age-appropriate control over behavior looks very different at ages 2, 4, and 8. It is important for those who care for young children to be aware of general differences related to age, as well as individual differences in development among children at the same chronological age. Behavior problems can sometimes be generated or increased by expecting too much or too little internal control for the developmental age of a particular child.

Summarizing previous research, Kopp (1982) suggests a developmental progression in the growth of self-regulation—from early "control and system organization" (including the control of arousal and sensory–motor modulation) that begins during the late prenatal period and the first 3 months after birth, to the development of "compliance" during the 9- to 12-month period, to the emergence of "impulse control" in the second year. Increasingly sophisticated forms of self-regulation develop from ages 3 or 4 onward. It is not clear, however, how these changes in self-regulation occur. Psychological theories provide accounts of development, but the accounts differ and are sometimes conflicting.

One area of conflict involves the degree to which the child spontaneously develops self-regulatory systems in everyday interaction with people and objects in the environment. To what extent is the child active in devising the means for control, and to what extent are these controls the result of external intervention? Does the child need specific coaching and training to learn self-regulation? Behavioral theories attribute the greatest amount of responsibility for development to explicit training, and Piaget's theory attributes the least.

Although the differences can be confusing, they must be considered carefully for several reasons. First, many of the differences among theories result in differing implications for what should be done to support development. Behavioral theory, for instance, suggests the need for a much more active and directive approach to intervention than Piaget proposed. Second, different theories consider quite different types and patterns of child behavior to be significant for development. In order to decide which behaviors to monitor and support, it is necessary to decide which theory or combination of theories is most relevant to particular age groups, particular areas of functioning, and particular situations. Finally, different theories can help the observer distinguish behavior patterns in children that had not been noticed before. A toddler's normal striving for independence, for instance, might otherwise be interpreted as stubbornness or defiance.

Many aspects of a child's functioning are *interrelated* in the development of self-regulation. Physical maturation and sensory–motor development are linked to the growth of control over emotional, social, and cognitive activities, and motivation influences the direction of development in all of these areas. Each area of functioning influences and is influenced by the others, making it difficult to consider them separately. Physical maturation and sensory–motor development, for instance, affect the possible types of physical activity, social interaction, and cognitive problem solving a child can attempt. On the other hand, physical activity, social interaction, and cognitive challenges influence a child's physical and sensory–motor development.

Cognitive and social development are also interrelated. Cognitive stimulation, and guidance in developing and applying problem-solving strategies, is typically presented to a child in the context of social interaction and is mediated through language and culture. The child's participation in social interaction and ability to understand social interaction, in turn, are influenced by cognitive development. In early childhood, social and cognitive processes are particularly intertwined and interdependent.

Motivation influences self-regulation in all areas of functioning. It gets physical, social, and cognitive activities started and keeps them going by providing both the direction or goal for action and the force necessary to sustain effort. Motivation is at the center of self-regulation and must be considered in relation to the development of all forms of voluntary control.

Another major issue and challenge for caregivers of young children is how to *support* the development of self-regulation. What kinds of supports are useful at what ages and in what situations? As is the case in defining and describing the development of self-regulation, there is some disagreement about the answers to these questions. Some stress the shaping role of the environment and advocate an approach based more on training and external reinforcement. Others emphasize the importance of the child's active discovery and construction of patterns, rules, and strategies for control. Both types of processes (patterning from the outside in and from the inside out) occur, but the relative weighting given to each, in general and at different ages, is critical for providing effective support for development.

Especially in early childhood, the nurturing of self-regulation requires an integrated approach that considers the "whole child." Young children cannot separate their feelings, thoughts, and actions as older children and adults learn to do. Their physical, social, emotional, cognitive, and motivational abilities and interests are intertwined. This means that support offered for self-regulation in the social or emotional area, for instance, has to be provided at a level appropriate to a child's physical, cognitive, and motivational development. It is also important that the child be able to control a function before control is required of her. Infants cannot stop crying on demand, and 2-year-olds are not able to consider the thoughts and feelings of others as 6- or 7-year-olds can.

This book reviews major theoretical perspectives and research evidence related to the development of conscious, voluntary self-regulation in young children from birth through primary school. It also proposes ways in which this information can provide guidelines for parents' and teachers' efforts to nurture the growth of self-regulation in young children. First, similarities and differences among various theories and research data are described in relation to the way self-regulation is defined, the way development is accounted for, and the types of influences and supports for development that are proposed. These similarities and differences are also discussed in relation to proposed applications of theory and research to practice, with suggestions about how the varying perspectives can be integrated or can provide complementary approaches to supporting the growth of self-regulation.

The book is divided into two parts. *Part I* describes the major theoretical and research perspectives on the nature of self-regulation and how it develops in different areas of functioning. Chapter 1 provides an overview of important theoretical perspectives on self-regulation in young children, including the psychoanalytic, behavioral, social learning, social cognitive, cognitive-developmental, and information-processing positions. The empirical research related to each of these perspectives is characterized. Chapters 2 through 6 examine the development of self-regulation in different areas of functioning. Chapter 2 focuses on the interrelation of motivational and self-regulatory processes and provides accounts of the ways in which motivation for control may develop. Chapter 3 reviews theory and research on how the child learns to control and direct emotions and their expression in behavior. Chapter 4 describes theory and research related to the development of prosocial and altruistic tendencies. Chapter 5 focuses on the development of "executive" or meta-cognitive control over attention and cognitive processing. Chapter 6 describes recent research on the development of control systems in the brain.

Part II integrates material from the preceding chapters and suggests practical applications. The development of self-regulation and methods of supporting it are described in three chapters, each focusing on one early childhood period: infancy to age 3, preschool and kindergarten, and the primary grades. In each of these chapters there are sections providing (1) an overview and synthesis of the theoretical and research material from Part I, which describes the development of self-regulation in the relevant age range and the effects of the environment on this development, and (2) a "research to practice" section that suggests ways of evaluating settings, caregiver behaviors, learning and teaching routines, and appropriate activities or tasks for each age group. Finally, in an epilogue, there is a brief review of missing pieces in the field and of the issues in child rearing and education raised by this book.

Part I

━━━━━━━

Theoretical and Research Perspectives on Self-Regulation

The six chapters in Part I examine theoretical and research perspectives on the development of self-regulation in young children and the importance of early experience. Chapter 1 reviews the major theoretical accounts of how self-regulation develops. It describes the psychoanalytic, behavioral, social learning, and social cognitive perspectives; the cognitive-developmental perspectives of Vygotsky, Piaget, and neo-Piagetian theorists; and the information-processing theory perspective. Chapters 2 through 6 focus on the development of self-regulation in specific areas of functioning. These include the development of motivation for self-regulation (Chapter 2), emotional and behavioral control (Chapter 3), interest and skill in directing behavior in prosocial ways (Chapter 4), the ability to control cognitive processing (Chapter 5), and the development of control systems in the brain (Chapter 6). In Chapters 2 through 6, theory and research associated with the development of self-regulation in target areas of functioning are described in relation to each of four age ranges in early childhood: infants, toddlers, preschool and kindergarten children, and primary school children. The importance of experience for each age range is discussed.

1

Overview of Theoretical Perspectives on Self-Regulation

Psychologists have described the nature and nurture of self-regulation in a variety of ways. In some cases different theories provide complementary models that focus on different areas of development, such as emotional or cognitive self-regulation. In other cases theorists propose alternative ways of defining self-regulation or accounting for its development in a single area. Often, a theoretical approach or position cannot be described in relation to a single theory because it includes a variety of theories within a general framework, as is the case with social cognitive theory and information processing theory. Sometimes a single theory generates an evolving theoretical and research tradition, such as the theories of Freud and Piaget have done. The learning theory or behavioral position has evolved over eighty years and includes a number of different theories.

In this overview, major theoretical perspectives relevant to self-regulation in young children are described and compared with alternate approaches. The theoretical positions examined are those proposed by selected psychoanalytic, behavioral, social learning, social cognitive, cognitive-developmental, and information-processing theorists. Individual theories within each tradition have been selected for inclusion in this overview because of their relevance to evolving perspectives on self-regulation.

THE PSYCHOANALYTIC PERSPECTIVE

Freud's theory focused on emotional development. He saw the development of self-regulation as an outgrowth of emotional needs and drives. In his model of the mind, the "ego" is the mental mechanism that is responsible for consciousness and the adaptive control of behavior. The ego serves the "id," which is the repository of basic drives and the energy for action. Id drives evolve with biological development in a series of "psychosexual stages" from infancy into adolescence. The ego must learn to gratify these drives in the real world in ways that will not offend the moral demands of society, internalized as the "superego" (Freud, 1923, 1930, 1965). From this perspective the primary developmental task for children is the development of a strong ego that is capable of controlling inappropriate impulses and coping effectively with reality to satisfy the requirements of both basic drives and social mores.

Freud proposed that individuals are born with a finite amount of psychic energy, residing initially in the id. This energy can be allocated to different parts of the mind (ego, superego) to cope with the demands of external reality and internal drives (id) and constraints (superego). Freud assumed that the goal of all activity is the reduction of psychic tension (a buildup of energy) that can come from a variety of sources: (1) biological changes (changing hormones, drives, and physical capacities), (2) external frustrations (from people, objects, or events that block the gratification of drives), (3) internal (psychic) conflicts between the different parts of the mind (id, ego, and superego), (4) personal inadequacies (inability to cope with external or internal demands), or (5) anxiety (fear of physical or psychological pain or loss) (Hall, 1954). The reduction of tension from any of these sources produces pleasure.

Freud saw human self-regulation as a struggle to keep the warring forces of the personality under control and to cope with their demands successfully in the real world. The ego is the relatively conscious and rational executive of the personality that organizes information from the internal and external environment and directs behavior. It emerges in infancy and gains strength throughout early childhood by acquiring increasing amounts of energy allocated from the reservoir in the id. The id invests more energy in the ego when the ego is successful in obtaining gratification or pleasure for the id in the real world. The superego is a primitive conscience, formed when the child's understanding of the constraints imposed by society are internalized at about the age of 6. From this point on the ego must satisfy the demands of the superego, as well as those of the id, in order to be successful and grow in strength (A. Freud, 1936). It must obtain pleasure in the real world to satisfy id drives, but must do so in ways that do not violate the social rules internalized in the superego.

Later "ego psychologists" in the psychoanalytic tradition reconceptualized the role of the ego, freeing it from subservience to id drives. Because it is the part of the mind that has the ability to learn and adapt, Hartmann (1958) characterized the mature ego as relatively independent from the id and possessing its own source of energy or motivation. Robert White (1959, 1960, 1963) proposed an inherent ego drive for competence, which has been incorporated into theory and research on "intrinsic motivation." White proposed that children (and adults) experience a feeling of competence when the ego adapts effectively to the environment. Erik Erikson (1959, 1963) added the notion that the ego develops a sense of "identity" (being a distinct individual) in the context of its interactions with the social world. Generally, ego psychologists characterize the ego as an active autonomous structure capable of meeting its own needs and striving for competence and identity. From this perspective the ego can be considered a relatively powerful and intrinsically motivated vehicle for self-regulation.

Because children do not have a mature ego, they are not considered as free of instinctual impulses and drives as adults. From the psychoanalytic perspective, self-regulation in children is increased as they develop ego strength. The ego is strengthened when it is successful in coping with external reality and satisfying id drives in the real world. A strong ego can channel and control id impulses and, after the superego is internalized, can reach goals in ways that conform to the rules of the culture.

The concept of ego strength as the power to cope with reality and curb impulses, and its proposed etiology in development, have implications for the development of self-regulation, which are discussed in Chapters 3 (on controlling emotion and behavior) and 4 (on engaging in prosocial behavior). White's description of the ego's need for a sense of competence is also considered in relation to intrinsic motivation for control in Chapter 2 (on the interrelation of motivation and self-regulation).

THE BEHAVIORAL PERSPECTIVE

Theorists in the behavioral tradition view self-regulation as learned self-control. This learning is largely attributable to factors external to the child, such as reward contingencies in the environment and explicit training. Building on Pavlov's (1927) early work, behavioral researchers have demonstrated the power of associative learning to "condition" automatic responses in both animals and humans. The work of Thorndike (1898, 1911), Hull (1943, 1952), and Skinner (1938, 1957, 1974) demonstrated the power of the consequences of behavior to shape its direction and frequency. Behavioral theorists have generally focused on the ways the external environment controls the behavior of individuals, rather than on the control exercised by them.

Self-control in this tradition has recently been defined as the choice of a larger but more delayed outcome and is contrasted with "impulsiveness," which is the choice of a smaller but less delayed outcome. Self-control is considered a function of the "relative size of and the relative delay of the outcome" (Logue, 1995, p. 9). Self-control also includes being able to use and control the behavior strategies needed to obtain rewards. Operant conditioning theory as outlined by B. F. Skinner (1948, 1974) has been used to teach self-control in a variety of situations (Graham, Harris, & Reid, 1992). Individuals are taught to select clear and appropriate goals that promise the largest reward available in the specific circumstances, to pay explicit attention to ("monitor") their own actions, to repeat specific learned instructions to themselves or consult lists of instructions, and to reward themselves in the short term in ways that are ultimately connected to long-term rewards in the external environment. The basic components of self-regulation, from the operant perspective, are goal setting, self-instructions, self-monitoring, and self-reinforcement.

From the perspective of behavioral theory, the development of self-regulation requires children to learn to assess the relative value of a variety of rewards, to learn to choose appropriate goals, to give themselves effective instructions or follow instructions provided, to monitor their own activities, and to reward themselves for behaviors that will ultimately be rewarded in the environment (or will keep them from being punished). The child's ability to judge the relative value of rewards, control impulsive behavior, and use effective strategies for obtaining rewards develops as a combined outcome of factors such as activity level (Siegman, 1961), cognitive abilities (Rodriguez, Mischel, & Shoda, 1989), maturation (Kopp, 1982), and learning (Mischel & Patterson, 1979). Learning can occur as a result of everyday experience in the environment or deliberate training. This means that the child's judgment and ability to control impulsive behavior changes with age and experience.

Experiences with real rewards in the environment contribute significantly to learned preferences. For instance, experiences of receiving adult approval may increase a child's interest in receiving this reward. Cultural norms and values, mediated through accidental or deliberate tuition from parents, teachers, peers, the media, and other sources, can also affect the child's valuing of rewards—both those previously experienced and those never experienced. For instance, a low or negative valuing of adult approval by peers can decrease the value of this reward for children. A high value placed on being a sports or media celebrity can increase the value of these rewards for young children although they may never have directly experienced them.

In addition to learning the relative values of specific rewards, children also learn about behavior control from both unplanned experiences and deliberate instruction or training. Experiences of receiving rewards after delays appear to help children learn to wait (Eisenberger & Adornetto, 1986). Experiences of receiving larger rewards after working hard for them appear to help children learn to value effort (Eisenberger & Adornetto, 1986; Eisenberger, Weier, Masterson, & Theis, 1989). Children can also devise or be taught specific strategies for increasing control over their own behavior (Mischel & Mischel, 1983; Mischel, Shoda, & Rodriguez, 1989). For older children these can include keeping track of one's own responses (self-monitoring) and administering one's own positive or negative consequences (self-reward or self-punishment) (Shapiro, 1984).

Generally, the view of self-regulation provided by behavioral learning theories focuses on how the child learns the relative value of rewards and how the child develops strategies for controlling responses in order to gain the most advantageous rewards.

THE SOCIAL LEARNING THEORY PERSPECTIVE

The first social learning theory (Dollard & Miller, 1941, 1950) grew out of an effort to combine the insights of Freud with the behavioral learning theories of Pavlov and Hull. Dollard and Miller wanted to "combine the vitality of psychoanalysis, the rigor of the natural-science laboratory, and the facts of culture" (1950, p. 3) and to explain how socialization occurs. In this early social learning theory, the child was assumed to be regulated internally by drives and habits and externally by the reward contingencies of the environment, much as Hull's theory had proposed. Imitation of others was added as a learned generalized strategy for directing behavior to obtain rewards.

In addition to including imitation as a strategy for guiding behavior, Dollard and Miller proposed that it was possible to use language to think through an experience step-by-step without needing to act it out and learn from mistakes. They suggested that language could be used as a form of verbal trial and error—talking through behavioral possibilities—which avoided the need for behavioral trial and error (Dollard & Miller, 1950). This model allowed a form of planning ahead, which increased (theoretically) the number of ways in which self-regulation could occur.

Albert Bandura (1977, 1997) transformed social learning theory by proposing that learning through observation occurs without the need for performance or reinforcement and by emphasizing the importance of cognition in observational learning. In this model self-evaluation plays a central role, both as a basis for motivation to self-regulate and as way to provide feedback for improving self-regulation attempts. Bandura suggests that the individual gains information about which behaviors are rewarded and valued in the environment (and which are not) by observing her own behaviors and the behaviors of others and evaluating their effects. These evaluations lead to the development of "expectancies" about the probable outcomes of specific behaviors, and the establishment of internal criteria ("performance standards") for judging the adequacy of the behaviors in specific contexts. The individual then uses performance standards to regulate her own behavior and to evaluate its effectiveness, and as a basis for self-reward (for "perceived self-efficacy") when the standards are met. Bandura's model of an intrinsically motivated self-regulatory system incorporates extrinsic rewards and punishments as "information" about the usefulness and effectiveness of behaviors in the environment. As performance standards are developed, ongoing behavior becomes regulated relatively more by these internal criteria and relatively less by external rewards and punishments.

From Bandura's theoretical perspective, the development of self-regulation in children requires the development of expectancies for the outcomes of behavior and performance standards for self-evaluation that are appropriate to the child's age, abilities, and level of experience or learning. Self-regulation that is adaptive in a particular situation depends first on the appropriateness of the child's expectancies for the outcomes of behavior in that setting. If a child has inappropriate or inaccurate expectations about the outcomes of behavior, she may not behave adaptively. The adequacy of self-regulation also depends on the appropriateness of the child's performance standards. If a child has standards that are too high, self-reward (for perceived self-efficacy) will be unlikely, because performance can not meet the standard. If performance standards are too low, the standard will be reached too easily and the level of performance attempted by the child may not match her potential.

Bandura proposes that behavior and thinking are "reciprocally determined" by models and events in the environment, the individual's own capabilities and behaviors, and her evaluation of both the environment and herself. A child or adult is self-regulated in a particular performance area to the degree that she has developed internalized performance standards and goals in that area that support independent self-guided activities (including learning activities) and provide criteria for self-evaluation and self-reward. Motivation is inseparable from cognition and action in this model.

THE SOCIAL COGNITIVE PERSPECTIVE

The area of study known as social cognition includes theories and research concerned with how children and adults understand themselves and others. The field combines elements of social, cognitive, and developmental psychology. Researchers interested in social cognition examine cognitive processing of social information. They study a wide range of topics, including the formation of social schemata (cognitive structures representing organized information about social concepts or persons), social inferences, social attitudes, and age-related changes in social perception and judgments. Bandura considers his social learning theory a social cognitive theory as well, because it focuses on the cognitive mediators of behavior. Topics in the area of social cognition that are particularly relevant to self-regulation include causal attribution (Rotter, 1966; Weiner, 1979) and perceived psychological control (Bandura, 1977; deCharms, 1968).

Social attribution theories are based on the premise that people are motivated to explain or make sense of their experiences because they have a cognitive need to organize and classify information in coherent and consistent ways. Theorists that focus on causal attribution (Heider, 1958; Kelley, 1967; Rotter, 1966; Weiner, 1979, 1986) assume that people are interested in understanding the causes of events, in order to predict the future and exert some degree of control over their own actions and the events and people in their environments.

Rotter (1966) proposed that there are stable differences in beliefs about the "locus of control" among individuals. He argued that some people, called "internals," believe that they have the ability to control the occurrence of reinforcing (rewarding) events; others, called "externals," believe that rewards are controlled by luck, chance, or powerful others. Weiner (1979, 1986) suggests a more complex model of causal attribution in which judgments are made about the "locus" of causes (internal or external to the individual), the stability of a behavior (how modifiable it is), and the controllability of future behaviors, events, and outcomes.

Causal attributions have been found to influence expectations for future actions and outcomes, emotions, and behavior. Internal locus of control has been associated with motivation and achievement in school (Phares, 1976), and research by Dweck and her colleagues suggests that children develop somewhat stable beliefs about their ability, or lack of ability ("learned helplessness") to cope with school tasks (Diener & Dweck, 1978; Dweck, 1975; Dweck & Repucci, 1973). Dweck (1975) notes that when children have failure experiences, only those who have been taught to attribute failure to a lack of effort persevere in the task.

Beliefs about the source of control in the environment are an important part of the causal inference process, but a sense of personal control is also integral to the self-concept and self-esteem (Bandura, 1977; deCharms, 1968; Hendrick, 1942; White, 1959). The perception of individual self-efficacy (Bandura, 1997) or "personal causation" (deCharms, 1984) motivates self-regulatory behavior and increased effort. When individuals feel able to control situations, they set realistic goals, determine actions they can take to reach the goals, and assess their progress toward reaching them (deCharms, 1976). Feelings of control and freedom are also related to responsibility (Brickman et al., 1982) and can reduce the experience of stress (Glass, Reim, & Singer, 1971).

Social cognitive theorists view children and adults as active information processors, engaged in constructing a coherent model of their social worlds. Research suggests that beliefs about control and effectiveness affect an individual's involvement in activities, the manner in which activities are carried out, and the amount of effort or persistence expended in the process (Bandura, 1982; Rotter, 1966; Schunk, 1989; Weiner, 1985).

THE VYGOTSKIAN PERSPECTIVE

Vygotsky (1962, 1978) emphasized the role of the social–cultural environment in shaping self-regulation, although he thought the desire for control is innate. He assumed that the child brings a desire to act effectively and independently and a capacity to develop higher-level mental functioning to her encounters with the culture (as experienced in interactions with others), but that goals and the means to reach them are culturally determined and learned. Beyond biologically determined tendencies shared with animals, humans learn what to want or value as well as the strategies required to obtain what is wanted, and both goals and goal-directed strategies may differ substantially across cultures.

Like Piaget, Vygotsky assumed that conflict promotes development. Using a "dialectical" model proposed by Hegel and Marx, he thought that change occurs by means of a thesis, antithesis, and synthesis process. The child tries to reconcile a currently held concept (thesis) to a new, different, or conflicting one encountered in social interaction (antithesis), by constructing a synthesis of the different ideas. The child is active in this process but does not act alone. She learns to think by constructing or "co-constructing" and internalizing progressively more adequate versions of the intellectual "tools" of the culture modeled or actively taught by more advanced others. Cultural tools include the psychological tools of language, writing, counting, art, and other symbolic aids to communication and thought.

Interactions that promote development may involve active "scaffolding" (Wood, Bruner, & Ross, 1976), "guided participation," or "building bridges" (Rogoff, 1990) on the part of an adult or a more experienced peer. The more experienced person assists the child by providing prompts, clues, modeling, questions, strategies, and other supports that allow the child to accomplish tasks she cannot yet accomplish independently. To be effective in promoting the development of the child's own independent, self-regulated action, this assistance must be provided in her "zone of proximal development," a hypothetical psychological area that represents the difference between what the child can already do independently and what she can do with help. The help provided should, optimally, be the minimum necessary for the child to construct the new understanding or skill (or synthesis) so that it does not interfere with developing independent self-regulation.

Vygotsky's notion of the zone of proximal development (ZPD) as readiness to learn, or the growing edge of competence, in any area of development is similar to Piaget's understanding of what is necessary for "equilibration"—a restoration of mental balance by resolving conflict—to occur. Equilibration can occur only when the conflict or discrepancy is "assimilatable" enough to be recognized by the child and her current mental structures are capable of adjusting ("accommodating") to the new information. In Vygotsky's view the child can advance only the width of her ZPD at any point in time. Social assistance or teaching outside this zone is presumed to be ineffective.

Although both Vygotsky and Piaget thought development proceeded when the child internalized her interactions with the world, Piaget emphasized the importance of the physical world of objects and Vygotsky focused on the social world. Vygotsky thought that both knowledge and the means for self-regulation are inherently social in origin. What are initially understandings mediated by and shared with other people, become internalized by the child and available for her own independent use. The child progresses from coregulation assisted by others to self-regulation using the tools acquired from others.

The psychological tools of a culture allow humans to move beyond the "elementary" mental processes we share with animals, such as involuntary attention and associative memory, to "higher level" mental processes such as voluntary attention and memory, abstract thinking, and voluntary self-regulation. Elementary mental processes are controlled by external stimuli and rewards. When individuals develop higher-level processes, they are able to use language and other symbolic tools to voluntarily control their own actions and thinking.

Vygotsky (1962) considered that the key psychological tool needed for human self-regulation is language. He saw language as the primary means through which culture is transmitted and the primary vehicle for thought and voluntary self-regulation. These language functions are developed in the child over time, and Vygotsky described stages in their development. He thought that language is used for self-expression and communication with others before it is used for regulating thought and action. He stressed the importance of egocentric or "private" speech, which was observed in young children by both Vygotsky and Piaget. Piaget (1926) noted that egocentric speech, in the form of repetition, "monologues" when the child was alone or "collective monologues" in the presence of others, was ineffective for communication. He considered it an immature form that vanishes when the child understands the needs of the listener and develops "socialized speech."

Vygotsky saw evidence of verbal commentaries on ongoing activities and self-instructions in the child's egocentric speech. He thought that this speech is intended for the self rather than others and that at first it follows or accompanies the child's ongoing activities. Later in development it precedes and assists or directs them. He thought that this "self-talk" or private speech is the child's primary means of voluntary self-regulation. It is overt in the beginning; then, at about the age of 6 or 7 (when Piaget also noted its disappearance), it "goes underground" and becomes internalized and indistinguishable from thinking itself. At this point language becomes the primary vehicle for both thought and self-regulation. There is a great deal of current interest in Vygotsky's understanding of the developmental progression and function of private speech, and an increasing body of research is supporting his position (Berk, 1994).

Vygotsky pointed to the importance of culture in the development of higher level thought and self-regulatory function, and researchers have been examining the cultural and contextual relatively of these processes (Bruner, 1990; Cole, 1992; Cole & Scribner, 1974; Luria, 1976; Rogoff, 1990; Schweder, 1991; Valsiner, 1988; Werch, 1985). Although human groups universally construct language and cultural tools, the specific tools vary, so people of different cultures may think and solve problems in different ways. A number of researchers have noted the powerful effects of schooling on the formation of the mind, especially Western schooling with its emphasis on the "decontextualization" of words, examining them and the systems of concepts they support as objects of study (Cole, 1990; Donaldson, 1978, 1987; Rogoff, 1990). Such decontextualization may assist children in developing a metacognitive awareness of their own thinking processes. Vygotsky thought that scientific thinking was one of the most valuable tools developed by modern society and that it developed in children in interaction with their teachers in schools.

THE PIAGETIAN PERSPECTIVE

As both a biologist and a developmental psychologist, Piaget considered self-regulation to be as intrinsic to the mind as homeostatic self-regulatory processes are to the body. He assumed that the purpose of mental self-regulatory processes is to allow optimal adaptation to the external environment, just as the purpose of homeostasis is to preserve an internal balance of biological processes sufficient to support life and growth.

In Piaget's model of cognitive adaptation, development occurs by means of two complementary processes. These "equilibration" processes allow information from the environment to enter and sometimes change existing cognitive structures. If incoming information matches or is similar enough to existing mental structures or "schemas," it is incorporated or "assimilated" into them. If incoming information is relevant to existing schemas but is inconsistent or conflicts with them, the structures are revised or alternate structures are constructed to "accommodate" the new information (Piaget, 1926,

1952). The processes through which adaptation and development occur (assimilation and accommodation) are the same and they are automatically self-regulating. As the child actively interacts with people
and objects in the environment, information from these interactions
that is not consonant with existing mental structures causes mental
conflict or "disequilibrium." This mental imbalance precipitates ac-
commodative changes in the schemas, and the child constructs increasingly adequate representations of reality (Piaget, 1985).

A variety of types of information may be presented to the child,
but the schemas incorporate only what her particular level of development allows. Piaget suggested that cognitive development occurs
in specific, qualitatively different stages based on both the types of
mental representations the child is capable of constructing and the
types of processing (mental "operations") the child uses during that
period. He proposed that these qualitative shifts in mental structures
and processing occur when the child is approximately 2, 7, and 12
(Piaget, 1954, 1967, 1970).

Infant thinking is considered action-based or "sensory–motor"
(Piaget, 1952). The child can learn to control only sensory–motor actions. At about age 2, she begins to be capable of symbolic "representations," which support both the development of language and
engagement in pretend activities (Piaget, 1926, 1962). The child can
control behavior in an increasing range of activities but is not yet capable of logical thinking and cannot control her own thought processes. She has not yet understood the difference between her own
thinking and the thinking of others and does not appreciate the psychological distinctions between humans, animals, and inanimate objects. A preschool or kindergarten child can increasingly control her
activities in order to stay within known constraints in the environment, but her thinking is relatively inflexible (not fully operational).
Centered in her own perspective, the child in this age range has a difficult time considering the rights and perspectives of others without
external guidance. She tends to focus on the static states of objects
rather than their transformations, and on appearances rather than
underlying realities. Piaget called this the "preoperational" period.

Toward the end of the early childhood period, at the age of 6 or
7, Piaget proposed another qualitative shift in the way the child
thinks. External actions become fully internalized in mental structures that are more flexible and, therefore, more "operational."

Thinking is less centered on one aspect of a problem or situation, and the child can remember transformations of objects and mentally reverse them. She is now capable of logical thinking about the concrete world she has experienced. She is also less egocentric and can consider the perspectives of others in making decisions. Piaget called this the "concrete operational" period. The child is capable of taking more independent responsibility for her own actions and can negotiate with others to define and create rules for social interactions. She is also interested in, and independently capable of, fairness and playing by the rules in games and in reality.

Piaget's final stage begins beyond early childhood at about the age of 12 (early adolescence). In this "formal operational" period the child's thinking capacities approximate those of an adult. It is not until this period that the child becomes capable of systematic scientific reasoning, propositional logic, and thinking hypothetically about worlds she has never experienced.

Both Piaget and Vygotsky considered scientific thinking the highest form of human thought. Piaget thought of the child as a little scientist engaged in forming hypotheses about the world and testing them in interaction with it. He believed that logical thinking could not be directly taught but had to be independently discovered and mentally constructed by the child. In contrast, Vygotsky thought that scientific thought is the result of human teaching—especially teaching in schools.

This difference in the way higher-level thinking processes are acquired also appears in the way Piaget and Vygotsky describe "universals" in human thought. Piaget thought that the capacity for logical and scientific thought is universal. Vygotsky thought that the capacity for language and culture is universal, but that without culture, the only thought processes all humans share are also shared with the higher animal species.

From Piaget's perspective, the direction of development is toward increasingly stable mental structures and processes that represent reality more adequately and are therefore more adaptive. The development of thinking is automatically regulated by the equilibration processes (assimilation and accommodation) as the child interacts with objects and people in her environment. Emotions exist but are given meaning and direction by thought (Piaget, 1967). Decisions and behavior are regulated by the child's cognitive capacities, and self-regulation increases quantitatively and qualitatively with cognitive development.

THE NEO-PIAGETIAN PERSPECTIVE

Piaget's theory generated a large body of research that attempted to test the accuracy of his descriptions of children's capacities at different stages of development (Flavell, 1971, 1986) and the generality of the stages across cultures (Cole, Gay, Glick, & Sharp, 1971; Cole & Scribner, 1974). More recently theorists have combined Piaget's proposal that children actively construct models of their environment, and show stage-like changes in thinking, with concepts from information-processing theory and with new information on the development of the brain.

Robbie Case (1985, 1992) and Kurt Fischer (1980; Fischer & Rose, 1994) suggest that stage-like changes in knowledge are domain specific, and that there appear to be general stages because children's information-processing capacities change with age. Younger children have more limited memory capacities, more limited control over attention, and fewer "executive control structures" (Case, 1992), as well as less knowledge and fewer skills in specific cognitive areas. Biological constraints imposed by different stages of brain development as well as differences in experience account for qualitative shifts in thinking.

THE INFORMATION-PROCESSING PERSPECTIVE

Information-processing theory is a framework of theories and research programs that use the computer as a metaphor for cognitive processing. Theorists and researchers build and test models of the ways attention, perception, and memory work together to process information about the environment, make decisions, and solve problems. Some use computer simulation to model human thought processes. Others use the computer metaphor and computer terminology—such as input, encoding, programs, processing, sensory "channels," memory "store," feedback, decision rules, and output—to describe human thinking. They measure processing time, errors, and loss of information in order to assess attention, perception and memory difficulties in tasks, and the difficulty of tasks as a whole.

Research in the information-processing framework combines a rigorous methodology with a new language for talking about mental processes. The computer metaphor has allowed researchers to talk about mental events in a way that allows integration of attention, perception, and memory in "flowchart" models that can be tested and revised. Self-regulation is described in terms of innate and learned programs that include and make use of "executive routines," rules, plans, and strategies, which allow the individual to regulate ongoing activities (Lezak, 1982; Miller, Galanter, & Pribram, 1960; Siegler, 1989; Siegler & Jenkins, 1989). Computer programs can use information in their memory banks or "stores," organize and reorganize internal and incoming information, follow a plan of action, select appropriate operations or strategies for specific problem situations, correct these operations by using feedback from the ongoing operations of the program, and ultimately produce some form of "output." Newer computer programs can even be designed to "learn"—to profit from their mistakes, "adapt" to a variety of problem situations, and become increasingly effective and efficient. Human brains have limited processing capacities in comparison with computers and do not appear to perform these processes in the same ways, but the computer analogy helps researchers think about how brains are different from computers and how they might be performing the same kinds of tasks.

Information-processing theories and research suggest that what develops in children is the capacity to engage in more organized, efficient, and effective cognitive processing. As they interact with people and objects in the world, they actively encode and organize information and actively make use of feedback to modify their own processing. With age (maturation and brain development) and experience children are able to encode the features of their environments more fully and effectively (Siegler, 1984; Sternberg, 1984), organize and retrieve it more effectively in memory, develop increasingly complex rules and strategies for processing and making decisions (Siegler, 1986, 1989), generate plans of action for problem solving (Cocking & Copple, 1987; Scholnick & Friedman, 1987), and monitor their ongoing activities, modifying the plan and strategies if necessary (Sternberg, 1984). Toward the end of the early childhood period (at about age 6 or 7), children also begin to develop metacognitive skills that allow them to understand, monitor, and control their own cognitive processes (Brown, 1978; Brown & DeLoache, 1978; Flavell, 1978). They gain better control of attention and memory and learn not only to make better use of feedback, but also to actively seek it to improve their performance. Development is considered continuous and linked to biological maturity and experiences rather than psychological stages.

Information-processing theorists assume that children are spontaneously curious about their environment and want to be successful in understanding and controlling it. Annette Karmiloff-Smith (1979, 1986) worked with Piaget and his colleagues and has reformulated many of Piaget's ideas in information processing terms. She is particularly interested in what drives development and has suggested that children are motivated to control their own processing. She differs with Piaget's proposal that it is primarily cognitive conflict that promotes cognitive growth and has proposed that children want to expand control of both the external environment and their own internal systems for dealing with it. Her research indicates that they will try to find ways of controlling situations even when such control is not necessary for problem solving.

SUMMARY

A variety of psychological theories include proposals about the mechanisms that mediate self-regulation and about how self-regulation develops during early childhood. This chapter has reviewed the psychoanalytic, behavioral, social learning, social cognitive, Vygotskian, Piagetian, neo-Piagetian, and information-processing perspectives. Table 1.1 compares these perspectives in regard to the sources or mechanisms for self-regulation and what causes its development over time.

Freud saw human self-regulation as a struggle to keep the warring forces of the personality under control and to cope with their demands successfully in the real world. He proposed that the ego is the source of developing control. Strength, in the form of energy, is given to the ego by the id insofar as it is successful in gaining gratification and avoiding punishing situations. Ego psychologists in the psycho-

TABLE 1.1. Sources of Self-Regulation and Causes of Development According to Different Psychological Theories

Theory	Source(s) of self-regulation	Cause(s) of development of self-regulation
Psycho-analytic	Ego deals with conflicting inner forces (id and superego), copes with the environment, and seeks "competence/efficacy"	Growth of ego strength from successful interactions with the environment and accompanying growth of self-esteem and self-confidence
Behavioral	Learned contingencies of reinforcement Learned ability to wait for delayed reinforcement Learned self-instruction strategies	Training in: • experiencing delayed reinforcement • giving self-reinforcement for delaying reinforcement • giving self-instructions • giving self-reinforcement for trying and for success
Social learning	Internalized performance standards (internalized representations of what constitutes competent or effective behavior) Self-evaluation—leading to self-reward (feelings of self-efficacy) if standards are met or self-punishment (feelings of self-contempt) if standards are not met	Learning performance standards from: • own performances and outcomes (reinforcement or punishment) of these • observing others and the outcomes of their behaviors Experiencing and observing reinforcement for self-regulated behaviors (leading to self-efficacy evaluation for self-regulation)
Social cognitive	Perceived ability to control events in the environment	Experiences of control Attribution of control to own actions and competence
Vygotskian	Innate curiosity and interest in independence	Private speech (internalized language that guides action and thought)
Piagetian	Equilibration—cognitive need to restore mental balance by resolving mental conflict or disequilibrium Interest in exploring and creating interesting effects in the environment	Cognitive development—increasing cognitive understanding of the physical and social environment and development of logical thinking (allowing increasingly adaptive and effective thinking and interactions with people and objects in the environment)
Neo-Piagetan	Innate interest in problem solving Domain-specific increases in control	Development of increased information-processing capacities that support independent problem solving and control Domain-specific increases in self-regulatory skill
Information processing	Innate interest in problem solving and control	Development of "executive" functions, including rules, plans, and strategies that support independent thought and action

analytic tradition suggested that the ego has energy of its own that provides an innate drive for competence and efficacy.

Theorists in the behavioral tradition view self-regulation as learned self-control. They consider that behaviors, including the internal behavior of thinking, are shaped by the reward and punishment contingencies in the environment. Children become self-regulated to the extent that they learn to wait for delayed reinforcements, give themselves (learned) instructions to guide behavior and problem solving, and learn to administer self-reinforcements for following these instructions.

Social learning theorists, notably Albert Bandura, consider self-regulation the result of internalized performance standards that guide behavior, and self-reinforcement or punishment according to whether or not these standards are met. Performance standards are derived partly from the individual's own history of being rewarded or punished for activities and partly from observations of the behaviors of others and their consequences. Self-reward (perceived self-efficacy) is the result of living up to performance standards. Self-punishment (self-contempt) is the result of failing to live up to these standards. Performance standards effectively guide behavior to the extent that they are appropriate for the individual's capacities and for the environment.

Social cognitive theorists focus on the importance of the individual's perception of the environment and her own effectiveness in it. They propose that there are relatively stable differences in people's beliefs about their causes of internal and external events and their own ability to control them. An individual's "attributions" about the cause and controllability of a situation influence her belief that she can control it and her willingness to attempt it.

Lev Vygotsky focused on the role of social and cultural factors in the development of thinking and self-regulation. He believed that the child is controlled by others initially, but that this control shifts to the child as she internalizes the mores of her culture and its symbolic tools. Language is the most important tool for self-regulation. The child learns to think and to give herself instructions using "private speech."

Piaget considered self-regulation an innate property of human cognitive adaptation. In his equilibration model the processes of assimilation (fitting new information into existing cognitive structures) and accommodation (modifying the structures to accommodate new information) are continuously involved in maintaining adaptive adjustment ("mobile equilibrium") to the environment. As cognitive structures incorporate an increasingly accurate understanding of the environment, the child is able to regulate behavior more effectively and efficiently within that environment. Piaget also described qualitative shifts, or stages, in the child's cognitive structures and the way she is able to think about the world and other people.

Neo-Piagetian theorists focus on domain-specific increases in skill and self-regulatory capacity. They often include concepts from information-processing theory and new information about the development of the brain, and focus more specifically on the development of attention, perception, and memory. They deemphasize Piaget's concept of generalized stages, considering these to be more the result of brain maturation and resulting changes in information-processing capacity.

Information-processing theories suggest models of human thinking and problem solving, using the computer as a metaphor for brain functioning. They try to model and describe the way attentional, perceptual, and memory processes work together to support thinking and problem solving. They describe self-regulatory processes in terms of executive routines, rules, strategies, and plans that are modified and improved with biological development and experience. Humans are considered capable of self-modification of the regulatory programs they use to guide behavior and thinking.

Each of these theoretical perspectives has influenced thinking about self-regulation in young children and generated some related research. The following four chapters in Part I examine theory and research that have contributed to our understanding of the role of motivation in self-regulation (Chapter 2) and how children learn to control emotions and behavior (Chapter 3), engage in prosocial behaviors (Chapter 4), and control their own cognitive processing (Chapter 5). Chapter 6 examines the contributions of recent research on the developing brain to our understanding of the development of self-regulation.

2

Interrelation of Motivation
and Self-Regulation

Motivation and self-regulation are so closely related that in practical situations they are virtually inseparable (Prawat, 1998). The *ability* to control actions and thoughts is conceptually separate from the *wish* to do so, but when voluntary self-regulation occurs in the natural environment, motivation is involved. Because the brain mechanisms that generate what we describe as motivation are intrinsic to both thought and action, our thoughts and preferences are colored by innate and learned emotional–motivational factors (LeDoux, 1996). Choices, decisions, and actions are influenced and often biased by them. Young children's choices and actions are especially affected by emotional–motivational coloring because they are less able to separate feelings from thoughts and behaviors. They are also less likely to reflect consciously before they act.

Motivation and self-regulation are intertwined in two major ways: (1) people are innately rewarded by competence and control (Hunt, 1963; Piaget, 1952; White, 1959), and (2) they need self-regulated control to reach other goals. Humans show spontaneous interest in controlling their own bodies, their actions in the environment, and their cognitive processing and problem solving. They also take spontaneous pleasure in influencing objects, people, and events in the environment. Simple engagement in some of these activities appears to be rewarding, and carrying them out with skill leads to feelings of competence (White, 1959) or self-efficacy (Bandura, 1997). People also become motivated to reach specific goals in the environment and to obtain other types of rewards, such as social approval and material gain. Self-regulation is usually required to achieve these goals and rewards.

Educators are becoming increasingly interested in self-regulated learning, behavior management, and motivation for these kinds of control (Biemiller & Meichenbaum, 1998; Zimmerman, Bonner, & Kovach, 1996). As learning is viewed less as a transfer of information provided by teachers and more as constructed understandings on the part of students, educators are searching for ways to promote motivation to engage in self-directed learning and problem solving. They consider this kind of motivation a prerequisite for independent learning, a mastery orientation in the classroom, and a persistent, planful pursuit of goals (Dweck, 1986; Harter, 1978). In addition, interest in self-regulation provides support for the lifelong learning that is currently being recommended for everyone in our fast-changing world.

Current controversies about the need for "structure" in education are also related to beliefs about motivation and control. Advocates of more flexible classroom organization and curriculum programs believe that children have both the competence and the need to make significant decisions about their own learning. They think that children are more likely to learn to control their own behaviors and to be effective problem solvers if they are given a considerable amount of choice and control over their learning activities and goals (Deci & Ryan, 1985, 1987). They also assume that interest in learning and feelings of competence are related to the capacity for pursuing one's own goals and interests. This approach is supported to some extent by developmental theories (Bruner, 1970; Piaget, 1952, 1954; White, 1959, 1960) and by "decision" and "attribution" theories, which describe how people assign causes for behavior and other events (deCharms, 1968, 1971; Deci, 1980; Rotter, 1966; Weiner, 1986). People who make causal attributions that are more internal and controllable are more interested in attempting to control their own activities and external events than those who believe that others or "fate" is in charge.

Advocates of standardized curriculum sequences and goals tend not to assume or rely on a child's innate interest in learning and self-regulation. They focus more on the power of the environment to shape motivation and self-control. Those in the behavioral tradition attempt to *produce* motivation for self-regulation through reinforcement. They reward instances of behavior control, focused and organized involvement in prescribed learning activities, and persistence until these activities are successfully completed (Logue, 1995). B. F. Skinner (1948) described a series of programmed steps that can be used to teach self-control to young children.

Social learning theorists stress the power of example. They describe how watching the behavior of others, and its rewarding or punishing consequences, organizes and motivates the behavior of the observer. Performance of an observed behavior is motivated partially by the observer's expectation of external reward or punishment, and partially by internal rewards or sanctions (Bandura, 1986, 1997; Zimmerman, 1989, 1995). Individuals are considered to develop internal standards of behavior from observing the consequences of their own and others' experiences. They then reward themselves with feelings of "self-efficacy" for living up to these standards, or punish themselves with "self-contempt" for failing to do so. Bandura (1997) considers these internal ("intrinsic") rewards and punishments more powerful than external consequences. Performance standards are derived from experience, however, and are shaped by the environment. From this theoretical perspective, the individual is less a seeker of control than one whose motivation and behavior are controlled ("reciprocally determined") by a combination of internalized standards and perceived external consequences.

Vygotsky (1962, 1978) believed that culture and language are the central elements in motivation and self-regulation. He was particularly interested in the power of social mediation and mentoring in the development of control (Berk & Winsler, 1995; Luria, 1961). He assumed that individuals have innate motivation for self-regulation and independent action, but that motivation to control specific situations and reach specific goals is acquired from others who transmit knowledge about which values and goals are approved by the culture. To a great extent the child learns what to want.

This chapter reviews evidence for intrinsic motivation for self-regulation and describes how it develops in tandem with experiences of control. It also discusses ways in which personal and cultural goals and values, and certain other environmental factors, influence its development.

INTRINSIC AND EXTRINSIC MOTIVATION

Intrinsic and extrinsic motivation have been distinguished by examining the sources of the rewards they provide (Pintrich & Schunk, 1996; Stipek, 1998). Intrinsic rewards are those that are internal to an individual or activity. A person may be rewarded by engaging in an activity for its own sake or by feelings of "competence" that the activity generates. For instance, a child (or an adult) may draw a picture because drawing is an enjoyable process or because seeing that she draws well is pleasant. She may throw a ball because throwing is fun or because watching the ball hit a target or go through a hoop leads to feelings of competence. She may follow rules in the classroom or in a game because she has internalized adherence to these rules as performance standards and can reward herself with feelings of competence or self-efficacy for living up to them.

Extrinsic rewards are external to the individual or the activity. A child may draw a picture to please a parent, read a book to conform to class expectations, or play a game to beat the competition. She may conform to external rules to win praise or avoid punishment from a parent or teacher.

In many situations both intrinsic and extrinsic motives are involved in an activity. A child may read a book because she enjoys reading *and* because it will be useful in a school project. She may play soccer for fun *and* to win social approval. She may conform to socially approved standards of behavior to please *both* herself and others. In many real-life situations extrinsic motivation complements intrinsic motivation. Achieving culturally approved goals, for instance, may enhance feelings of competence. However, in some situations extrinsic rewards can undermine intrinsic motives (Deci & Ryan, 1987; Lepper, 1981). When extrinsic rewards change the overall purpose or goal of an activity from achieving personal satisfaction to earning external rewards, intrinsic motivation can diminish or disappear. If a child who loves swimming is consistently encouraged to enter swimming competitions, rewarded with praise and prizes for winning, and receives expressions of disappointment or criticism for a less-than-first-place finish, intrinsic enjoyment in the activity may be reduced. The child may want to swim only in competitions and only in those she has a good chance of winning.

Whether motivation to engage in an activity is relatively intrinsic or extrinsic depends on the person involved, the nature of the activity, and the context in which it occurs. The same activity can be intrinsically motivating for some children and extrinsically motivating for others. In addition, a child who enjoys an activity, such as reading, can be intrinsically motivated to engage in it in one setting, such as at home, and extrinsically motivated to read in a school context where the teacher offers a gold star for each book read.

MOTIVATION FOR SELF-REGULATION

Self-regulation can be an intrinsically motivated activity in itself. Intrinsic motivation for self-regulation can be described as a generalized tendency to be rewarded by, and then seek mastery or control of, the self, others, or the physical and conceptual environment. Infants show delight in both physical and cognitive mastery as early as the first 3 months of life (Bruner, 1970; Papousek, 1967; Piaget, 1952). They work to control their own bodies, influence other people, and gain increasing cognitive mastery of the world around them. Children as young as 1 or 2 years of age are also clearly motivated to choose their own activities and to direct and control the way these activities are carried out (Ames, Ilg, & Haber, 1982; Erikson, 1963), and people of all ages are interested in independent action and problem solving.

Self-regulation is required or assumed in other motives that are considered intrinsic. Motivation for competence, for instance, requires some degree of control as a condition for satisfaction. In order to experience a feeling of competence, it is necessary to feel responsible for the actions or outcomes that demonstrate competence.

Self-regulation is also required for successful engagement in a large number of activities, whether they are intrinsically or extrinsically motivated. A child needs internal control of both behavior and cognitive processing to do a puzzle, build a block tower, or engage in dramatic play with peers, regardless of why she wants to do these things.

Motivation for Self-Regulation in Infants

From early infancy children appear to be rewarded by controlling their own activities and producing effects in the environment. They take pleasure in controlling interesting sights and sounds and work persistently to produce them (Bruner, 1970; Piaget, 1952; White, 1959). Motivation theorists have proposed an inherent generalized need for what has been called "competence," "effectance," or "mastery," which requires both self-direction and control over outcomes (Deci & Ryan, 1985; Dweck, 1986; Harter, 1978, 1981; White, 1959). In addition, developmental theorists have suggested that children are innately interested in independence and self-regulation (Inhelder & Piaget, 1964; Piaget, 1952, 1967; Vygotsky, 1962, 1978).

Infants (as well as adults) also seem to be innately rewarded by cognitive consistency and coherence. This includes pleasure in both recognizing familiar people, objects, events, and sequences and anticipating or predicting their appearance (Kagan, 1971, 1997; Piaget, 1985). They appear to be comforted or rewarded by familiar patterns and sequences and upset by too much novelty or discrepancy. Even infants want to know what is coming next. The tendency to notice, then search for consistency and prediction is important for the development of self-regulation because recognition of regularity is an essential prerequisite for the exercise of voluntary control.

Interest in Recognition and Prediction

Psychologists have often observed that people are interested in, and tend to seek, cognitive coherence and consistency. In the first half of the 20th century, Gestalt theorists proposed that the human mind spontaneously organizes incoming perceptual information in order to make it more orderly, meaningful, and similar to past experiences than it actually is (Koffka, 1935; Kohler, 1947, 1959, 1969). Bartlett (1932) suggested that memory operates in much the same way, mapping new information onto previously organized stores (schemas) in ways that make it more consistent with preexisting memories. He showed that people often distort or eliminate ("forget" or fail to store) discrepant or conflicting information. More recent studies (Greenwald, 1980; Loftus & Palmer, 1974) have supported these early theories.

A number of theorists have pointed to a need for cognitive consistency in adults. Leon Festinger (1957, 1964a, 1964b), a pioneer decision theorist in the 1940s, proposed a theory of "cognitive dissonance" to account for both consistency and change in beliefs and values. He found that incoming information that was not consistent with presently held views was unpleasant to people. They would attempt to "reduce the dissonance" either by failing to take fair account of the inconsistent information, ignoring or distorting it, or by changing their beliefs and values in order to accommodate it. The need for consistency was such that once a person had decided to stay with an old position or had changed to a new one, she tended to exaggerate the evidence in favor of the decision and against the opposing point of view. Festinger found that once a position was held or an activity continued in the face of opposition or "insufficient rewards," its value for the individual was *increased* and that organisms—from rat to man—"came to love that for which they had suffered" (1964b, p. 537). These findings contrast with the behaviorist view that reduced or insufficient reinforcement leads to the reduction or "extinction" of a response. Cognitive dissonance theory generated a large number of subsequent studies, and most appear to support Festinger's contention that inconsistency between beliefs and behaviors is emotionally arousing and leads to efforts to resolve the discrepancy (Cooper & Fazio, 1984).

Schachter (Schachter & Singer, 1962) extended the need for cognitive coherence to the interpretation of emotions. He suggested that most emotional states are merely conditions of physiological arousal which require a label, and that labeling results from an "evaluative need." In his experiments subjects were given an arousal-producing drug, whose effects they did not know, and were placed in a room with a stooge who was instructed to behave in an angry or giddy way. The subjects were highly susceptible to emotional reactions parallel to those of the stooge and tended to label their subjective feelings in line with the other person's action pattern. Schachter proposed the following:

> 1—Given a state of physiological arousal for which an individual has no immediate explanation, he will label this state and describe his feelings in terms of the cognitions available to him. To the extent that cognitive factors are potent determiners of emotional states, it could be

anticipated that precisely the same state of physiological arousal could be labeled joy or fury or jealously or any of a great diversity of emotional labels depending on the cognitive aspects of the situation.

2—Given a state of physiological arousal for which an individual has a completely appropriate explanation (e.g., "I feel this way because I have just received an injection of adrenaline") no evaluative need will arise and the individual is unlikely to label his feelings in terms of the alternative cognitions available. (1962, p. 299)

Schachter's model, like Festinger's, viewed uncertainty as unpleasant.

Berlyne (1960) conceived of all directed thinking as motivated by conceptual conflict and, thus, uncertainty. As a theorist in the behavioral tradition, he thought that conceptual conflict or uncertainty led to a drive-like state that required resolution. Doubt, perplexity, contradiction, conceptual incongruity, confusion, and irrelevance are instances of the kind of conceptual conflict that generates motivation for directed thinking. Berlyne's concept of thinking for the purpose of resolving conflict is similar in some ways to Piaget's proposed need for cognitive equilibrium (1985). Piaget's view, however, assumes a mind actively engaged in trying to understand its environment that actively seeks contact with the world outside itself. Berlyne's concept of "epistemic curiosity" or "the drive to know" considers curiosity to be the result of present or projected future conflict situations and is therefore more reactive in nature.

Jerome Kagan (1971) proposed a "motive to resolve uncertainty" that is similar to Festinger's dissonance reduction and Berlyne's conflict resolution motivation. He considered that this motive is activated by incompatibility between cognitive structures and either experience or behavior. Sources of uncertainty are "discrepant events" that do not fit expectancies, inconsistency or lack of congruence between two ideas or between an idea and a behavior, and inability to predict the future. Kagan suggested that emotions such as distress, anxiety, fear, shame, or guilt may occur if no appropriate responses are available to resolve uncertainty.

More recent work has focused on a need for consistency in the self-concept or "self-schema" (Markus, 1977; Markus & Nurius, 1986; Swann, 1983, 1985; Tesser, 1988). The self-concept is a model that organizes perceptions of the self in a variety of situations (Harter, 1983). It makes the past coherent and allows us to form expectancies for our actions and abilities in the future. It is important that this self-model or schemata be relatively consistent; therefore, we find discrepant feedback upsetting. Research suggests that we try to surround ourselves with people and situations that will verify our own view of ourselves (Swann, 1983). If we have a high estimate of ourselves and our abilities, we seek friends and colleagues who confirm this self-evaluation. If we have low self-esteem or consider that we have little competence in a certain area, we tend to interact with people who evaluate us in a similar way.

Early Interest in Recognition and Prediction. In addition to theory and research on the unpleasant effects of uncertainty, there is ample evidence that recognition and prediction produce positive affect, even in very young children. Infants appear to be innately rewarded by recognition of patterns in the environment and the ability to anticipate events (Hunt, 1996; Jensen, 1998; Piaget, 1952; White, 1959). From the earliest months they smile at familiar people, objects, and events and begin to notice the regularities in the environment. They stop crying in anticipation of being comforted or fed when they perceive the approach of the caregiver and show surprise when there are changes in expected sequences (Bower, 1977).

Piaget (1952) suggested that the young infant's smile indicates pleasure in recognition apart from and even before its social function. He describes this pleasure in his own children:

> Examination of our three children has left us no doubt that the smile is primarily a reaction to familiar images, to what has already been seen, inasmuch as familiar objects reappear suddenly and release emotion, or again inasmuch as a certain spectacle gives rise to immediate repetition. It is only very gradually that people monopolize the smile precisely insofar as they constitute familiar objects most inclined to this kind of reappearance and repetition. But in the beginning, anything at all can give rise the emotional recognition which elicits the smile. (p. 72)

Kagan and his students proposed that smiling occurs not so much in response to mere repetition as to an "effortful act of recognition" (Super, Kagan, Morrison, Haith, & Werffenback, 1972). They observed the visual attention, smiling, vocalizations, and heart rate of 5-month-old infants to hanging mobiles of varying degrees of familiarity. They found that both attention and positive affect were highest in response to stimuli in the middle range of familiarity—that is, familiar stimuli with slight variations or "discrepancies"—when the infant had to exert mental effort to recognize the stimuli.

Outside the laboratory situation infants reveal their pleasure in recognizing and anticipating events by smiling and vocalizing when engaged in familiar play routines. They show surprise when a familiar sequence does not follow the expected pattern and may become distressed if the sequence is interrupted or the violation of pattern is too discrepant (McCall & Kagan, 1970). As the child becomes familiar with the environment, she notices and is interested in novelty, as long as it is not too different from what is already recognized. There appear to be optimal levels of difference (or "incongruity" [Hunt, 1966] or "discrepancy" [Kagan, 1971; McCall & Kagan, 1970]) from the familiar that are attractive and interesting to children. If a stimulus or sequence is too familiar, it is no longer interesting; if it is too different, it may be frightening.

The notion that optimal levels of novelty are interesting and stimulating is supported by a variety of studies investigating the effects of various levels of stimulation and arousal (Fiske & Maddi, 1961; Helson, 1964; Kagan, 1997). Although there are individual differences, the most pleasant levels are typically in the medium range, with too much arousal producing negative emotions, including anxiety and fear, and too little producing boredom. Studies of fear in infants and young primates (as well as other animals) seem to support some form of the optimal variety notion. Too little novelty in the environment produces boredom, apathy, and self-stimulatory behavior. Novelty up to a certain level of difference from past experience produces exploratory behavior and apparent curiosity. Beyond that level (different for individuals with different temperaments and experiences) novelty produces fear.

Innate tendencies, such as temperament, may influence a child's preference for higher or lower levels of stimulation and for novelty, but experience—in calmer or more rowdy environments, for instance—also influences the child's expectations and adjustment over time. In addition, children are more interested in novelty in familiar rather than strange environments. It is interesting that, in most cases, negative affect and fear appear only after expectancies have been established. There seem to be a few innate fear responses to certain types of stimuli, such as loud noises and falling, but the fear of novel or strange objects, people, or events occurs only after recognition and familiarity have been achieved.

J. McVicker Hunt (1966) suggested that pleasure in recognition is the starting point for pleasure in predicting. He proposes roughly three stages of interest in the environment during the first 2 years of a child's life.

> During the first stage, the infant can be said to be attentive and responsive to changes in ongoing inputs. During the second phase he shows the beginning of intentions directed toward keeping or gaining perceptual contact with sources of input which have just become recognizable through repeated encounters. At the third stage, the child becomes interested in novelty: it is now that the principle of optimal incongruity becomes clearly operative. (p. 232)

Infants also demonstrate pleasure in anticipation and prediction. Hanus Papousek (1967, 1969) found that infants as young as 2, 3, and 4 months seemed to enjoy the problem solving involved in his head-turning experiments. They were rewarded with milk when they turned their heads back and forth in certain sequences. They appeared to develop "strategies" in response to the reward contingencies, and if the signals were not congruent with these strategies or expectancies, the infants usually showed signs of displeasure or distress. They also tended to smile and vocalize when their "solutions" proved correct. Many infants continued to respond even after they had their fill of the mild reward and refused it. Papousek concluded that infants have an innate ability to detect certain rules in environmental events and experience pleasure from their successful predictions and from successfully creating desired effects.

Piaget (1926, 1950, 1952, 1954) documented the young child's increasingly active interaction with the environment. He suggested that this interaction is accompanied by the generation of increasingly accurate hypotheses about the way the world works. In his view, interest in understanding the environment, and in constructing models of reality, develops as the child begins to interact with the social and physical environment and becomes stronger with experience.

Recent research suggests that the brain is designed to detect regularities and patterns and to connect events that occur in sequence, making causal inferences under some conditions (Dennis, 1991; Donaldson, 1987; Gelman & Kalish, 1993; Sylwester, 1995). From the beginning of sensory awareness, the baby notices recurring events and begins to build expectancies that will form the basis of internal control and self-directed attempts to control the external environment. As experience accumulates, increasingly useful and accurate patterns, categories, and rules are generated in relation to the surrounding environment and culture.

Interest in Control

A substantial body of theory and research underlines adult interest in self-determination and "being a cause" (deCharms, 1968, 1971; Deci, 1980; Deci & Ryan, 1985, 1987, 1991; Rotter, 1966). People are intrinsically motivated to choose their own activities and goals and feel more competent when they feel self-determined (Deci & Ryan, 1985). We tend to lose interest in activities and goals that are externally imposed and require external rewards to motivate continued engagement.

Adults are also rewarded by feelings of self-efficacy and control (Bandura, 1997; Rotter, 1966; Weiner, 1985, 1986). We experience pleasure in the perception of competence and control and are motivated to achieve it. We experience distress, depression, and feelings of helplessness when we feel out of control or unable to cope with environmental circumstances and may give up trying (Hiroto & Seligman, 1975). We are especially vulnerable to these negative outcomes when we attribute our lack of control to internal and unchangeable causes (Weiner, 1986).

Early Interest in Control. Infants also show spontaneous interest in the world around them, exploring first with eyes, ears, and mouth, then increasingly with hands and the rest of their bodies. The infant's attraction to new or complex visual stimuli has been documented many times (Bower, 1977; Fantz, 1964, 1965, 1967), and auditory and tactile input seem to be similarly attractive. Bruner (1969b, 1970) argued that the environment acts as an incentive to the development of complex skill learning and control by containing innately captivating "goals" (objects, persons, contingent events) that automatically elicit what he called "intention" in infants. His observations of young babies learning to reach and grasp convinced him that intention precedes and directs action through feedback and provides a criterion for terminating an act. This theoretical sequence of development—from intention to response—differs from both the classic behaviorist (response to reinforcement) sequence and the Piagetian theory that proposes an opposite development—from response to intention. In Bruner's view the child can "want" something she sees in the environment before she has experienced having it. The importance and mediating function of distance receptors (eyes and ears) in this scheme is again in contrast to the sequence theorized by Piaget, who proposed a sensory–motor or learning-based-on-action model.

Young infants show spontaneous interest in controlling their own motor movements and pleasure in influencing objects and people in their environment (Bruner, 1968, 1969a; Hunt, 1963, 1965; Papousek, 1967, 1969; Piaget, 1952). They persistently practice developing motor skills, working to bring movements such as head lifting, rolling, sitting, crawling, and walking under their own control (Ames et al., 1982; Gesell & Ames, 1974). They spend many hours reaching for objects, grasping small things, dropping and retrieving objects, and practicing countless other activities without encouragement and without reward.

Infants soon learn to create interesting effects in the environment and to make interesting sights last longer. A number of psychologists (Piaget, 1952; Rovee-Collier, 1989; Watson, 1966) have described children's early contingency awareness and their interest in creating effects in the environment. Piaget (1952) noticed an early delight in producing effects in his own three children:

> Lucienne, at four months, is lying in her bassinet. I hang a doll over her feet which immediately sets in motion the series of shakes [that had moved the doll before] . . . Her feet reach the doll right away and give it a violent movement which Lucienne surveys with delight. Afterwards she looks at her motionless feet for a second, then recommences. (p. 159)

> Jacqueline, at five months, looks at a doll attached to a string which is stretched from the hood to the handle of the bassinet. The doll is at approximately the same level as the child's feet. Jacqueline moves her feet and finally strikes the doll with a movement she immediately

notices. . . . The feet move, first without conscious coordination, then certainly by circular reaction. The activity of the feet grows increasingly regular whereas Jacqueline's eyes are fixed on the doll. (pp. 159–160)

At three months, after Laurent has learned to grasp what he sees, I place the string which is attached to the rattle in his right hand, merely unrolling it a little so that he may grasp it better. For a moment nothing happens, but at the first shake due to chance movements of his hand, the reaction is immediate: Laurent starts when looking at the rattle and then violently strikes his right hand alone, as if he felt the resistance and the effect. The operation lasts fully a quarter of an hour during which Laurent emits peals of laughter. The phenomenon is all the more clear because, the string being slack, the child must stretch his arm sufficiently and put the right amount of effort into it. (p. 162)

John Watson (1966) charted the development of "contingency awareness" in his own child at 2 to 3 months of age. He thought that the infant's contingency, or cause-and-effect, learning difficulties during the first 3 or 4 months were the result of immature memory span capacities, which put a severe time constraint on contingency awareness. To overcome this problem, Watson devised an artificial contingency, which consisted of performing a response that was visually rewarding to the child whenever the child visually fixated on the appropriate rewarding hand. The infant not only learned the contingency in three sessions (one a day) at the age of 2.2 months, he even more quickly learned a second and third contingency discrimination, showing apparent "transfer" from the original learning situation. Watson noted that the child also began to look for and discover other "natural" contingencies in his environment, and to attempt to manipulate them.

Other evidence of the young infant's ability to make use of artificially structured contingency situations comes from Bruner's (1968, 1969b) experiments with the sucking response. He found that it was possible to vary the sucking patterns of 10- to 17-week-old infants by differentially reinforcing mouthing or biting components of the child's natural pattern. Infants of these ages were also able and "motivated" to use nonnutritive sucking to suck a visual stimulus into focus if this artificial cause–effect sequence was arranged.

More recent studies (Gulya, Rovee-Colleir, Galluccio, & Wilk, 1998; Rovee-Collier, 1989) have shown that 3- to 6-month-old infants quickly learn to make mobiles move and bounce by kicking their legs when a ribbon is loosely tied to an ankle to allow this control. They kick vigorously and clearly enjoy manipulating the mobiles. The 1998 study also demonstrated that babies this young can learn and remember the order in which different mobiles are presented to them. Their ability to recognize regularity in an ordered sequence suggests that infants are capable of forming expectancies at a very early age.

A number of psychologists have also proposed an early and spontaneous interest in autonomy and effectiveness (Deci, 1980; Hendrick, 1942; Ryan, 1993; White, 1959, 1960). Their work suggests that children's early experiences with the environment teach them not only about objects and events in the world, but also about their own ability to cope with and influence them.

Robert White's (1959, 1960) theory proposes that the ability to predict regularity in the environment develops in interaction with increasing interest in affecting the environment, and that this creates a sense of "competence" in the individual. White's concept of competence subsumes the whole realm of learned behavior that the child comes to use to deal effectively with the environment. It includes locomotion, manipulation, skilled actions, language, and the growth of effective behavior in relation to other people. Noting that acquisitions of competence are made by young animals and children partly through exploration and manipulative play when drives such as hunger are in abeyance, White believed that the directed persistence of such behaviors warrants the assumption of a motivation independent of the traditional notion of "drives." He labeled this urge "effectance" or "competence" motivation and proposed that it has its immediate satisfaction or "reward" in a feeling of efficacy and its adaptive significance in the growth of competence in the environment. The child's *actual* competence and growing *feelings* of competence are built from her history of successful and unsuccessful efforts in the environment.

The Effects of Early Experience

There is a variety of evidence that environmental circumstances can serve to reinforce or damp interest in self-regulation. As suggested, young infants show spontaneous pleasure in recognition, prediction, and control; however, for specific motivation to develop and grow, the environment must provide circumstances that allow them to have these experiences. People, objects, and events must appear with enough regularity that they are recognized. Patterns and sequenced events must recur with enough regularity that they can be expected and predicted. People and objects must be sufficiently responsive to the infant's vocal and nonvocal signals that she discovers her power to have an effect on them. In uninteresting, confusing, or unresponsive environments this kind of motivation may not develop or may be weak and unfocused.

Although infants spontaneously attempt control of their motor movements and attend to their surroundings with all their sensory faculties, even these activities can be delayed in severely impoverished social and physical environments (Carlson & Earls, 1998; Frank, Klass, Earls, & Eisenberg, 1996). The social environment appears to be particularly important. Physical contact, sensitive social stimulation, and responsiveness to an infants's signals contribute to feelings of security (Ainsworth, Bell, & Stayton, 1972). These feelings appear to support the development of confidence or "trust" (Erikson, 1953, 1963), and competence motivation (White, 1959, 1960) that fosters effective engagement with the social and physical environment.

Experiments in "learned helplessness" in both animal and human subjects underscore the dependence of coping behavior on past experiences. Seligman (Maier & Seligman, 1976; Seligman, 1975, 1991; Seligman & Maier, 1967) found that experiences of unavoidable punishment made subjects stop trying to escape aversive circumstances. They appeared to learn that they were helpless (had no ability to control events) and passively accepted a variety of unpleasant or punishing situations.

The physical environment is also important. When the child's environment is either sterile and lacking in opportunities for interesting sensory experiences, or overstimulating or chaotic, her engagement with that environment may be delayed. A child who has not discovered interesting objects or events in the environment cannot learn how to look for and attend to them. A child who is confused or overwhelmed by overstimulation or chaos may find it difficult to focus and explore.

Patty Greenfield (1971) explored the implications of Jerome Bruner's (1969b, 1970) theory about the role played by goals in organizing behavior. She suggested two types of environmental circumstances that result in impaired "means–end relationships" (or goal-directed behavior) in young children. In one case, goal attainment is constantly frustrated, which leads to a "feeling of powerlessness," to a "shifting of responsibility outward," and to a "gambling approach to problem solving." In the second case, the environment can fail to provide a "growth-promoting sequence" of goals. Greenfield emphasized the role of the mother (primary caregiver) in structuring goal sequences, providing positive feedback, and reinforcing the child's feelings of competence.

A number of theorists suggest that experiences of competence in predicting and controlling various aspects of the environment promote increased interest in prediction and control, and increased confidence and skill in attempting to do so (deCharms, 1968; Harter, 1978; Rotter, 1966; White, 1959). Studies with animals (Seligman, 1975; Seligman & Maier, 1967), elementary school children (Dweck & Goetz, 1978), and adults (Hiroto, 1974) have shown that the lack of ability to control a situation leads to a belief that control is impossible. The expectation that control is impossible (or failure to learn that it is possible) reduces (or fails to support the development of) future attempts to influence or learn to control similar situations. When a perceived lack of control extends to many areas of functioning, the individual may abandon efforts to develop self-directed coping skills in the belief that what happens to her is controlled by luck, fate, or powerful others (deCharms, 1968; Rotter, 1966).

Both theory and research suggest that children's early experiences with people and objects influence the direction and strength of their motivation to control their own activities and to understand and influence the environment. When a young child has experiences in which she is able to recognize and predict events in her environment, she develops expectations that the world is coherent and that she will be able to understand it. When a child has experiences in which she is able to influence or control events in her environment, she develops an expectation that she will be able to direct her own activities effectively within it.

Motivation for Self-Regulation in Young Children beyond Infancy

Although motivation for self-regulation, or the capacity to be rewarded by self-regulatory functions, appears to be innate, most of the

specific goals that require and shape the development of self-organization and self-direction are derived from the environment. All children
are motivated to control their own physical and cognitive activities, to
control physical objects and events outside themselves, and to effectively influence other people, but the goals of action and thought and
the form and direction of social influence attempts are shaped by the
environment. In addition, both the motivation for control and the
child's self-regulatory goals change with age and experience.

As skill in self-regulation and control over internal capacities increase, the child acts on and learns to manipulate, influence, and control the external social and physical environment. Experience and
active experimentation also allow her to create and carry out increasingly adequate strategies and plans in order to reach goals (DeLoach
& Brown, 1987; Kreitler & Kreitler, 1987). She learns to choose
goals, to plan and organize activities in order to reach them, to monitor and control mental and physical behaviors mobilized to carry out
plans, and to correct or revise efforts that are not succeeding. If the
child's efforts succeed often enough and are rewarding, motivation to
attempt self-directed activities increases. With practice, the desire and
capacity to choose realistic goals, to plan effectively, to organize and
monitor thought and behavior, to correct mistakes and persist, and
ultimately to succeed in reaching planned goals, improve (Scholnick
& Friedman, 1987).

The child's developing interest and skill in self-control, and in
choosing and reaching goals in the social and physical environment,
can be encouraged or discouraged by the environment in which development occurs (Haste, 1987; McGillicuddy-Delisi, Delisi, Flaugher, & Sigel, 1987; Pasnak & Howe, 1993; Zimmerman & Schunk,
1989). The social and physical environment provides scaffolds for
the child's developing understanding and behavior. The reliability,
predictability, and responsiveness of the people in the child's world
and the physical objects the child encounters can have a major impact on the timing and direction of self-regulation (Dennis, 1991;
Kopp, 1982; Paris & Byrnes, 1989).

During the first 3 years support for the development of self-
regulation is focused on the types of experiences provided in the external environment and on the types of caregiver nurture and guidance that support intrinsic interest in self-regulation, the development of early impulse control, and awareness of goals (Kopp, 1982).

During the preschool years the emphasis is on encouraging the development of self-guidance, on providing opportunities to practice developing organized, self-directed action in social and task (mastery) situations, and on assisting (or "scaffolding") expanding self-regulatory skills in ways that support growing independence (DeLoach & Brown, 1987; Haste, 1987; Light, 1987; Scholnick & Friedman, 1987). During the primary school years the focus is on providing experiences that bring self-regulatory skills to the child's conscious awareness, so that she can reflect on alternative methods of self-control and self-direction and choose more effective ones (Barkley, 1997; Delisi, 1987; Donaldson, 1978).

Toddlers

Motivation for self-regulation and self-direction strengthens during the toddler years, which is one reason why this period is referred to as the "terrible twos" (Gesell, 1928). The toddler's urge for independence, or "initiative" (Erikson, 1963), is marked. Between the ages of 1 and 3 children increasingly want to do things themselves rather than having others make decisions or do things for them (Ames & Ilg, 1976; Ames et al., 1982). They are increasingly aware of the possibility of their control over themselves and their activities and increasingly want and demand it. However, they have not learned clearly what they can and cannot do, according to external rules or their own level of skill, and may often be frustrated in trying to reach goals because of external control or their own lack of competence (Nucci, Killen, & Smetana, 1996). Their inexperience may make their efforts to achieve control difficult for those around them, but children's strong striving for independence and mastery marks this period as significant for the development of self-regulation. What happens during these years can significantly advance, or cause difficulties in, the child's progress toward self-control.

In the social area, toddlers are interested in doing what others do. They watch other people and are increasingly able to internalize and imitate actions and words (Piaget, 1962). In addition to engaging in direct imitation, they can observe behavior, remember it, and display it at a later time. Internalized representations of the behavior sequences of others can become templates for children's regulation of their own behavior.

As children notice and remember more of the regularities in their environment and are more capable of moving around and manipulating things, they are increasingly motivated to tinker with the relationships they observe and attempt to predict and control them (Hunt, 1960, 1963, 1966; Piaget, 1952, 1954; White, 1959). Toddlers want their world to be orderly and predictable, and they want to be able to influence it. Piaget (1952, 1954) suggested that children's intrinsic motivation to understand the environment is powered by an innate need to avoid cognitive conflict (or "disequilibrium"). He proposed that this motivation is universal to all ages.

Children spontaneously form categories (Gelman & Kalish, 1993, 1998) as part of their innate propensity to cognitively organize their experiences. Perhaps this is because the brain spontaneously connects events that are perceived to be similar (since overlapping sets of neural networks are involved in perceiving them) (Gazzaniga, 1992). As toddlers acquire language, they also show great interest in putting people, animals, and objects into named categories. They ask the names of things they have not seen before, or generalize from past experience and apply a label they think fits. A chicken, observed for the first time, may be called a duck if ducks are familiar (a known category). The child's growing cognitive organization of the environment, assisted by the mastery of language, sets the stage for later control of cognitive processes (Berk, 1992, 1994; Vygotsky, 1962). As the child grows older, the relationship between cognitive organization and self-regulation becomes clearer, and the importance of this organization for effective self-direction becomes increasingly apparent.

Importance of Experience. The cognitive developmental literature and information on the developing brain suggest that later experiences build on earlier ones, and that patterns of functioning laid down during the early years provide the basis for later accomplishments (Shore, 1997). Motivation develops in a similar way. As children experience pleasure in understanding and mastery of the environment and their own self-control and self-direction, motivation to have these experiences increases. As they continue to experience pleasure from their success in these areas, children more actively seek opportunities to exercise and increase their developing skills.

Burton White's (1972) study of the development of competence in preschool children convinced him that the second year of life is particularly important. This is a time when mobility and burgeoning attempts to explore and master the environment challenge the caregiver's time and patience and require an understanding of the child's needs. White stresses the importance of programming the environment, providing developmentally appropriate materials to foster the child's autonomous play, demonstrating reinforcing (rather than restrictive) attitudes toward the child's independence and mastery attempts, and mediating effective language skills. Other studies (Ainsworth et al., 1972; Bronson, 1973; Crockenberg, Jackson, & Langrock, 1996; Nucci et al., 1996) also emphasize the importance of the caregiver's role in supporting autonomy and competence.

Preschool and Kindergarten Children

Preschool and kindergarten children move from a basic interest in exploring and affecting their environments to more focused motivation to reach specific goals (goal-directed mastery) (Hunt, 1960, 1965; White, 1959). Younger children in this age range may be more interested in the process of reaching a goal than in the final product. They may start out to paint a "dinosaur" and be satisfied to label their completed work a "house" if it looks like a house. Kindergarten children begin to have standards for judging their products. They are likely to tear up a drawing or knock down a block building that does not meet their expectations.

Psychologists have attempted to account for this transition. Heckhausen (1968) built a theoretical bridge between effectance motivation and achievement motivation. He viewed "pleasure from the effect" as a form of "self-reinforcement" that becomes contingent on meeting certain standards. According to this model, the child strives to master certain levels of difficulty in activities that involve competition or comparison with a standard of excellence. As children develop awareness of their own goals and intentions, "what had previously been mere pleasure from effects in the environment becomes now pride in own success; and prior displeasure from nonappearance of looked-for effects becomes now a feeling of shame because of failure" (p. 131).

Harter (1975, 1978) extended Robert White's (1959) "effectance" model by including a "desire to solve cognitively challenging problems for gratification inherent in discovering the solution" (1995, p. 370). She suggested that children can develop a preference for challenge, a desire to work for the gratification inherent in success, and internal criteria for success. Heckhausen (1968), achievement motivation theorists (McClelland, Atkinson, Clark, & Lowell, 1953), and social learning theorists (Bandura, 1977, 1997) also proposed that internal criteria for success mediate efficacy motivation and support self-regulation. The child (or adult) regulates her own behavior by comparing it with internalized representations or norms of performance and is motivated to meet or exceed the standard. Standards for performance begin to be developed during the preschool and kindergarten period as the child's interest gradually shifts from process only to both process and product.

Mastery motivation in young children has been defined as a "psychological force that stimulates an individual to attempt independently in a focused and persistent manner, to solve a problem or master a skill or task which is at least moderately challenging for him or her" (Morgan, Harmon, & Maslin-Cole, 1990, p. 319). Hauser-Cram (1998) noted that key components of this definition include attempts to master a task independently of adult direction, persistence in the face of difficulty, and selection of tasks that are neither too easy nor too difficult for the child. This parallels definitions of "achievement motivation" in adults (Atkinson, 1957; McClelland, Atkinson, Clark, & Lowell, 1953).

Importance of Experience. Research shows that the possibility of choice, perceived competence, and perceived control affect motivation (Deci & Ryan, 1985, 1987; Ryan & Grolnick, 1986; Swann & Pittman, 1977). Motivation for mastery or achievement is reduced or eliminated when the individual feels controlled by others (Deci, 1980; Dweck & Elliott, 1983). High levels of adult direction appear to reduce children's motivation to succeed with tasks on their own (Hauser-Cram, 1998; Morgan, Maslin-Cole, Biringer, & Harmon, 1991).

The perception of responsibility (control) and the ability to choose are essential for the arousal of mastery motivation in younger children and achievement motivation in older children and adults (who have more clearly defined goals and internalized standards of excellence for comparison). Individuals with high motivation to achieve choose tasks with intermediate levels of difficulty and risk—

not so easy that feelings of achievement will not be experienced, and not so difficult that achievement will be unlikely (Atkinson, 1957; McClelland, 1966). This choice is personal, because tasks present different levels of difficulty for different individuals. In preschool children, mastery motivation is aroused when a task is at least moderately challenging for the particular child (Redding, Morgan, & Harmon, 1988). When children are not allowed appropriate choices in tasks, or when their progress is unnecessarily controlled by adults or peers, motivation for mastery may be reduced or eliminated.

Coherence in the environment may also be important for the development of motivation for self-regulation and mastery. An understanding of goals and the internalization of standards of performance require an environment that supports these cognitive advances. Minuchin (1971) found that children who live in home conditions that are highly disorganized and unpredictable are less curious and less apt to explore the environment. Their conceptual grasp of order in the physical environment and of the relationships among objects is low. Order and predictability in the environment may support motivation for self-regulation as well as cognitive understanding.

Primary School Children

As children mature, the generalized need to feel competent differentiates into motivation for competence and achievement in specific areas, such as academics, sports, or crafts (Deci & Porak, 1978). Children may *become* motivated to engage in and improve their controlled performance in activities that they discover they can do well. Upon finding that they are "good at" throwing a ball, making friends, or reading stories, they may become interested in doing these things more often and working to increase their skill and control.

Zimmerman (1989) proposes that in elementary school, "students can be described as self-regulated to the degree that they are metacognitively, motivationally, and behaviorally active participants in their own learning process" (p. 4). Paris and Ayres (1994) suggest that what is missing from this definition is the purpose, direction, and force of the student's effort. They emphasize the importance of making choices or selecting goals, and that self-regulated learners can choose appropriate goals such as working toward mastery and task completion, or social cooperation, depending on the situation. "They know how to plan, allocate resources, seek help, evaluate their own performance, and revise and correct their own work" (p. 28). They are also intrinsically motivated, preferring tasks with choice, challenge, and control (Stipek, 1993).

During the early elementary school years children are also developing standards for judging the adequacy of their achievements (Zimmerman et al., 1996; Zimmerman & Schunk, 1989). Elementary school practices can have important effects on children's attitudes toward their own competence—and toward school and learning—during this period. They can also have major effects on motivation.

Feelings of competence, generated by experiences of success in mastering challenging tasks, increase motivation to engage in these activities. Children who believe they are academically competent are more interested in school learning activities (Harter, 1981, 1992). A sense of personal control also supports intrinsic motivation (Deci & Ryan, 1985, 1987), and self-regulated learning activities give students a sense of personal control (Zimmerman, 1985, 1995). External control, and rewards or punishments that enforce external control, have detrimental effects on intrinsic motivation and on self-directed learning (Lepper, 1981). Lepper and his colleagues (Lepper, 1981, 1983; Lepper & Greene, 1978; Lepper & Hodell, 1989) propose that this can be accounted for by an "overjustification" effect related to cognitive dissonance. When an individual is externally rewarded, she feels extrinsically motivated and controlled and is more likely to consider the task as a means to an end (external rewards) rather than an end in itself (with internal or intrinsic rewards). When an individual works in the absence of extrinsic rewards, she attributes motivation to her own interests.

External control and external rewards also diminish responsibility for the outcomes of learning tasks. When responsibility for success cannot be assigned or determined, results may be attributed to powerful others or to chance (deCharms, 1968, 1971; Rotter, 1966; Rotter, Seaman & Liverant, 1962). School-age children can also exhibit patterns of "learned helplessness" when they believe that they have little control over the events that affect them. They attribute their successes to external factors like luck and their failures to internal factors such as ability (Dweck & Elliott, 1983). Dweck (1986) also found that school-age "mastery-oriented" children seek challenge and are persistent in their attempts to solve difficult problems. Those who feel "helpless" avoid challenges and are less persistent.

Importance of Experience. Early elementary school experiences may be particularly important in determining whether motivation for self-regulated learning and achievement is strengthened, and incorporated into children's attitudes toward themselves and toward learning, or whether they begin to feel helpless. Children between the ages of 5 and 7 are beginning to judge not only the adequacy of the products they produce (in relation to their original goals), but their own adequacy. As they become increasingly self-aware, they begin to compare themselves with their peers and their skills with the skills of others.

Teaching strategies that compare children in ways that produce winners and losers may make children feel inadequate and helpless. Using external methods of control, providing rewards and punishments that are controlling, such as threats and deadlines, and the types of evaluation and surveillance that imply external control are also detrimental (Deci & Ryan, 1987). During this vulnerable period when self-consciousness is beginning, positive experiences may be especially valuable for preserving and nourishing mastery motivation, and negative experiences may be especially destructive.

SUMMARY

Motivation and self-regulation are highly interrelated. Self-directed learning, problem solving, and action can occur only when the ability to control thinking or behavior is accompanied by the wish to do so. Educators are becoming increasingly interested in promoting both self-regulation and the motivation for self-control and self-directed learning.

There is a convincing body of evidence that humans have intrinsic motivation for self-regulation. Very young infants appear to rewarded by controlling their own activities, interacting with people and objects in the environment, recognizing and predicting events, and influencing or controlling their social and physical world. Under favorable conditions, the child moves from having a relatively passive capacity for being rewarded by these experiences to actively seeking them. Infants move from a general responsiveness to incoming stimuli to active exploration, manipulation, and curiosity. Motivation to recognize and predict progresses from innate pleasure in recognition to an increasingly active interest in understanding the human and physical world. Motivation to influence or control progresses from an apparently innate joy in being a cause to an active interest in mastery and achievement as the child grows older.

Motivation for self-regulation may be particularly vulnerable to environmental influences. The cumulative effects of experience on this cognitively mediated motivation are more powerful than the effects of experience on visceral drives (for food, sleep, etc.). The environment provides goals and teaches the child about her own ability to reach them. A reasonable amount of order, regularity, and responsiveness in the environment allows the child to develop a sense that the world is predictable and influencable. Self-directed and successful interactions with the social and physical world support the child's feelings of competence and control.

Different kinds of environmental supports become important as the child matures. Infants need experiences that support their interest in exploration and experimentation and allow them to be successful causal agents. Toddlers need support for their burgeoning interest in independence and self-direction which allows them to experience some degree of success in their efforts. Preschool and kindergarten children need the kind of support for their developing self-regulatory capacities and interest in goal-directed mastery that strengthens their feelings of competence and control. Early elementary school children need experiences that build confidence and support their feelings of self-worth as they become increasingly self-aware and have a growing tendency to compare themselves with others. Children of all ages need an environment that is coherent and predictable enough to invite and reward their efforts at exploration and mastery at each level of development.

Intrinsic cognitive motives, such as motivation for self-regulation, are flexible and nonspecific. This results in both adaptive strength and vulnerability in development. Adaptive strength comes from the mind's ability to be interested in, and learn to know and cope with, a wide variety of physical and social environments. Vulnerability comes from the mind's dependence on the environment for stimulation, coherence (so it can learn to recognize and predict), and responsiveness (so it can learn to influence and control).

Table 2.1 summarizes the development of motivation for self-regulation in the four age ranges and the major effects of the environment on development at each age.

TABLE 2.1. The Development of Motivation for Self-Regulation and Effects of the Environment on This Development

Motivation for coherence, consistency, predictability	Motivation for competence, mastery, control	Effects of the environment
Infants		
Smile at familiar people, objects, and events Notice regularities and show pleasure in anticipating regularities Interested in assimilable novelty Spontaneously explore environment with eyes, ears, and developing motor activities	Work to control own body movements and develop motor skills Show pleasure in producing effects by own actions Show spontaneous interest in autonomy and effectiveness	Chaotic, overstimulating, or understimulating environments impede development Lack of ability to influence or control self, others, objects, or events impedes development and may lead to expectation of inability to influence or control
Toddlers		
Active interest in regularity and repetition, "order," and coherence (wants words repeated verbatim, things put in the same places, and activities done in the same ways) Active interest in exploring the environment	Strong push for independent action and control of own activities Strong push for control of decision making Beginning of interest in mastery activities Interest in imitation to master the activities of others	Coherence in the environment supports development Environment that allows choice and independence and is influenceable/controllable supports development Positive and responsive guidance of adults that supports independence strivings of toddlers supports development of motivation
Prekindergarten and kindergarten		
Active (though not necessarily conscious) hypothesis generation and experimenting Active efforts to understand using words (Why? How? Who? When? etc.) and actions Active effort to organize and classify perceptual environment	Increasing ability to choose goals effectively Increasing interest and persistence in reaching goals (mastery motivation) Developing internal criteria for judging success in reaching goals and pride in own success (active interest in social and mastery "competence")	Coherence and predictability in the environment supports understanding of goals, constraints, and standards of performance Opportunities for choice among tasks with appropriate levels of challenge (matching age and ability) support intrinsic motivation Experiences of effort followed by success increase perception of competence and control, and motivation to engage in similar activities
Primary school		
Increasingly conscious awareness of consistencies and predictability in the environment (and awareness of discrepancies) Increasingly differentiated understanding of the requirements of tasks Developing internal standards for performance and awareness of skills of others, which leads to increased self-judgment of own performance and skills in different areas	Increasingly conscious purpose (goal orientation and persistence), self-direction and control of action and thought (more capable of conscious self-regulated learning) Area-specific awareness of own competence influences interest and engagement in activities in these specific areas Perception of external control decreases motivation	Appropriateness of levels of challenge in the environment (for individual interests and skills) influences feelings of competence and motivation for mastery Opportunities for choice and control increase perception of control and interest in activity Negative judgments of others decrease feelings of competence and control Rewards and punishments external to the task decrease intrinsic motivation

3

Controlling Emotion and Behavior

Controlling arousal and the expression of emotions is an important part of self-regulated functioning. Psychologists have defined emotional control in two major ways: (1) as the capacity to regulate arousal appropriately in order to reach goals and (2) as the ability to control the behavioral expression of emotions in socially adaptive ways. Studies have linked emotionality to temperament, and differences in emotional expression to differences in self-regulation (Derryberry & Rothbart, 1988; Larsen, Diener, & Cropanzano, 1987; Thomas & Chess, 1977). Parenting practices (Eisenberg, Fabes, Schaller, Carlo, & Miller, 1991; Hardy, Power, & Jaedicke, 1993; Kochanska, 1991, 1993), peer interaction (Barkley, 1997; Furman & Masters, 1980), and experiencing stressful events (Compas, 1987; Sandler, Tein, & West, 1994) also appear to make a difference.

A large body of research by Nancy Eisenberg and her colleagues has related emotional self-regulation to social competence, and the lack of adequate control to behavior problems (Eisenberg & Fabes, 1992; Eisenberg et al., 1991, 1995, 1996). Others have shown that social competence is associated with behavior control (Block & Block, 1980) and low levels of problem behavior (Caspi, 1998). Early self-control is also related to later control. Attentional and behavioral control at age 4 or 6, for instance, is associated with appropriate behavior and social competence in school at age 8 (Eisenberg et al., 1997). In addition, there is evidence of increasing stability in emotional control over all of childhood and even the life span (Sroufe, Carlson, & Shulman, 1993; Urban, Carlson, Egeland, & Sroufe, 1991).

The development of control over behavior and the expression of emotions has been explained in different ways by different theories. In the psychoanalytic tradition the development of impulse control has been related to the development of a strong ego (Block & Block, 1980). In the behavioral tradition the growth of emotional control has been linked to learned strategies for controlling impulses (Logue, 1995). Cognitive developmental theorists have associated the control of emotions and behavior with overall cognitive development, including the decline of "egocentrism" (Piaget, 1962; Piaget & Inhelder, 1969), and the use of language for self-direction (Vygotsky, 1962, 1978). Information-processing theorists have related the development of "executive" control in all areas to the development of central processes, such as memory, and more adequate processing strategies (Case, 1985; Dodge, 1986; Garber, Braafladt, & Zeman, 1991). This chapter integrates theory and research to provide an overview of the development of emotional and behavioral control.

INTERRELATION OF EMOTIONAL, SOCIAL, AND COGNITIVE CONTROL

Theory and research suggest that emotional and behavioral control are related to both cognitive and social development (Sroufe, 1995; Thompson, 1990). Cognitive understanding and expectations determine emotional responses to some extent. Emotional arousal can be variously labeled (Lazarus, 1966; Schachter & Singer, 1962). Emotional responses can also be generated by our cognitive interpretations of the meanings of events. For example, the appearance of a face in a window can produce joy, fear, anger, or a range of other emotions, depending on the individual's cognitive assessment of the context and meaning of the appearance. Sroufe (1995) describes affect and cognition as "two aspects of the same process" (p. 117), and Piaget (1962) suggests that there is no such thing as a purely cognitive or purely affective state, since both are involved in all activity of the mind and each influences the other. Research on brain function shows that emotions are intrinsic to human information processing and that cognitively mediated "meaning" both interprets and generates emotional arousal (LeDoux, 1996; Schore, 1994; Shore, 1997).

The control of emotional expression and behavior requires an understanding of environmental constraints, the self-regulatory ability to exercise control, and the motivation to do so. Cognitive development is required for the child to learn to recognize, interpret, and remember her own emotions and to recognize constraints on their expression in the environment. Both maturation and experience are involved in producing the ability to exercise control, and both cognition and affect (in the form of motivation) are required for the child to actually exercise control.

Social development is also inextricably linked to the development of self-regulation. Although there are some innate mechanisms for the regulation of arousal (Kopp, 1982) and innate "temperament" appears to make a difference (Plomin, 1990), experiences with the social and physical environment provide direction (goals), constraints (rules), and practice in the adaptive expression and modulation of emotions and behavior. The child learns not only what to expect in the environment, but how she is expected to, or can successfully, respond and interact within it. Experiences with objects provide information about how to interact successfully with the physical world. Experiences with people provide support, models, and active guidance in how to interact successfully and appropriately with others. The child's sociocultural milieu provides the "cultural tool kit" of meanings and methods that guide and support cognitive growth, the development of self-regulation, and adaptation to the total environment (Bruner, 1986, 1990).

The development of self-regulation is so strongly linked with the social environment that it has been described as a gradual shift from "other control" (or dyadic regulation) to self-control (Schaffer, 1996; Sroufe, 1988, 1995). Although the child is active in developing her own self-regulatory capacities, she does not and cannot do this in isolation. She is supported and guided by caregivers and by culture. Sroufe (1989) suggests that the roots of self-regulation of emotions lie in the patterns of dyadic regulation with caregivers. Through reciprocal interactions with others the child develops a beginning awareness of the self as a separate individual. As she internalizes social values and is more able to control herself, she becomes able to engage in a more "responsive partnership" (Sroufe, 1995, p. 151) and gradually acquires the capacity to function independently.

Early experience appears to be formative as well as supportive in the development of emotional control. New research on the neurochemistry of the developing brain suggests that emotional events such as attentive mothering or stress can have major long-lasting effects on mood and behavior (Mlot, 1998; Schore, 1994). Sroufe (1995) suggests three other ways in which early experience is important. First, early successful adaptation produces resources for the child to draw on in later interactions with the environment. Second, individuals to some extent create their own experiences ("are both the artist and the painting," p. 156); previous learning influences what children will attempt and how they will attempt it. Third, current experiences are interpreted within the "frameworks" created by previous experiences. Children who have experienced primarily accepting and loving relationships view the intent of others in a more positive light than children who have experienced a large amount of criticism or rejection.

THE DEVELOPMENT OF EMOTIONAL
AND BEHAVIORAL CONTROL

In the rest of this chapter, issues related to the development of emotional and behavioral self-regulation are discussed in relation to each of four age groups: infants, toddlers, preschool and kindergarten children, and primary school children. The types of control available to each age range, the relation of developing control to both cognitive and social development, and the importance of the environment in facilitating the development of control at each age level are reviewed and discussed. The review focuses on differences associated with maturation or the environment, rather than innate differences such as temperament. Because genetic differences in emotional reactivity develop in interaction with caregiver and environmental differences and appear to be modified by external circumstances even in the development of the brain, the relative contributions of nature and nurture are difficult to disentangle (Sroufe, 1995).

The best-known overview of early phases in the development of self-initiated regulation of emotions and actions is that proposed by

Claire Kopp (1982). In the first phase, called neurophysiological modulation, innate physiological mechanisms protect the young infant from too much stimulation or arousal. During the first 3 months infants also protect themselves by turning away from sources of stimulation and by self-soothing activities such as sucking. In the next phase (sensorimotor modulation) infants become capable of voluntary actions that change in response to changes in the environment. They can voluntarily make contact with objects and people, and they learn to differentiate their own actions from those of others.

During the period from about 9 to 12 months, Kopp suggests, that babies begin to become capable of responding to external control. As they become consciously aware and capable of intentional, goal-directed action, they can begin to comply with external signals and commands. As they increasingly differentiate the self from others, they are more able to recognize what their caregiver wants and respond to it. It is during this period that active guidance from caregivers begins to be relevant in the development of precursors to self-control.

Kopp proposes that the child becomes capable of impulse control during the second year, with the assistance of emerging language, the development of strategies for tension reduction, and caregiver sensitivity to the child's needs and individual characteristics. She suggests that true self-control does not emerge until the preschool years (ages 3 to 4). During this phase the child becomes capable of complying with others' requests and behaving appropriately in the absence of external monitoring. These advances are possible because children of this age are cognitively capable of representational thought (recalling objects and images in memory) and understand that their own identity and the identities of caregivers continue over time (so caregiver wishes continue and actions have consequences). According to Kopp, self-regulation is different from self-control in degree but not in kind. Self-regulation merely involves wider-ranging central control mechanisms and greater flexibility in adapting to changes.

The integrated nature of development is clear from Kopp's overview. Physiological, cognitive, social, and emotional/motivational factors interact and exert reciprocal influences on all aspects of development, including the development of self-regulation. The child's capabilities and behaviors emerge from and reflect these developing inner patterns of organization. As changes in one area occur, they are integrated with and influence development in other areas. The child's experiences, mediated by the social and physical environment, therefore affect the whole child and influence development in all areas.

EMOTIONAL AND BEHAVIORAL CONTROL IN INFANTS

From the earliest months of life the child begins to adapt innate regulatory systems to the environment and develop internal control mechanisms that allow self-directed voluntary action. Sroufe (1995) notes that during the first 6 months the infant moves from general "affective states" to more specific emotional reactions. She develops an increasingly active role in regulating her own state of arousal, partly by more active involvement in producing stimulation. She also moves from global/diffuse to more specific/coordinated actions as a result of increasing "sensory, sensorimotor, and sensoriaffective integration," which Sroufe calls the roots of control (1995, p. 46). He comments:

> The tendency to impose order on experience is ever present. When order can be attained from novelty, incongruity (Berlyne, 1969), or uncertainty (Kagan, 1971), through mastery or repetition (Piaget, 1962), there commonly is positive affect; when the orderly flow of cognition or behavior is inalterably interrupted (Mandler, 1975), there often is negative affect. (p. 48)

During the first 3 months the infant is aroused by internal factors, such as hunger or discomfort, and certain external stimuli, such as interesting sights, sounds, and motions. She is soothed by the cessation of hunger or discomfort and by external stimuli such as holding and rocking or the sight, sound, or smell of the primary caregiver. "Heartbeat" sounds and the mother's voice are particularly effective, perhaps because these sounds were heard most clearly before birth. The infant uses gaze to maintain, terminate, or avoid social or other stimuli by looking toward or away from the source of stimulation.

In the period between 3 and 12 months the child is capable of engaging in voluntary action. She has an expanding repertoire of actions and social responses and can initiate them in response to people, objects, and events in the environment. Kopp (1982) calls this developmental advance "sensorimotor modulation" and notes that it does not involve "consciousness, prior intention, or awareness of the meaning of a situation" (p. 203).

During this period the baby watches and explores more actively. With increasing mobility and improving motor control the child is progressively more self-directed, moving away from the primarily reactive pattern of the younger infant. She is able to seek social stimulation and attention and interaction with objects, as well as respond to them, and to act on the environment more deliberately, exploring and experimenting (Bower, 1977).

Sroufe (1995) suggests that infants' emotional reactions are becoming more differentiated and more "idiosyncratic" during this period, as they are increasingly based on past experience. Infants begin to respond to context and learned meanings rather than isolated stimuli. They also acquire organized systems of emotions and behavior in which one reaction leads to another in meaningful sequences.

Emotional self-regulation is related to developing behavior control (Kopp, 1992). In the 3- to 12-month period children expand their techniques for regulating emotion (Rothbart, Ziaie, & O'Boyle, 1992) and are more able to both soothe and stimulate themselves. They begin to use more active ways of disengaging attention to soothe themselves, turning or moving their bodies away as well as looking away. Other self-soothing techniques include touching the head, putting the hand or thumb in the mouth, hand-clasping, and arm, leg, or body movements. In the second half of the first year infants are less likely to use diffuse arm, leg, or body movements to soothe themselves, and more likely to push an unwanted stimulus away or move away from it and toward the caregiver. Children in this age range are also more active in seeking stimulation. They reach out to, and ultimately move their bodies toward, objects and people. They also look around their environments more deliberately, searching for objects and people of interest.

In addition to the modulation of arousal and emotions, Kopp (1982) suggests, infants become capable of simple compliance with external control toward the end of the first year (9 to 12 months). They can begin to respond to warning signals and carry out simple one-step action requests such as waving "bye-bye" or moving toward a caregiver when called. Kopp believes that infants are now consciously aware and capable of some "intentionality" and goal-directed behavior. As infants are able to differentiate themselves from others, remember what caregivers want, and exhibit or inhibit certain behaviors, the caregiver assumes a greater role in fostering the development of precursors to self-control such as compliance.

Importance of Experience

A large part of human emotion is related to social interaction and develops in social contexts (Fogel, 1993), and early development appears to be particularly important. Recent research on the developing brain suggests that infants need affectionate, responsive, reliable, and predictable care for emotional, social, and cognitive development (Shore, 1997). Such care makes the child feel secure and supports the development of attachment to a primary caregiver. The mother helps the child set daily rhythms and sleep–wake cycles both before and after birth (Hofer, 1988). Social interactions and routines also help the child regulate arousal by providing appropriate stimulation when the child is awake and alert and soothing routines that precede periods of rest or sleep (Als, 1978).

The child's early social environment and the development of attachment also appear to affect later self-regulatory functions. Nurturant and responsive early care is related to fewer behavior problems in the face of stress (Egeland, Carlson, & Sroufe, 1993), and lack of such care is associated with impaired emotional regulation (Perry, 1996; Sroufe, 1989). There also appears to be a link between poor attachment, and aggression and violence (Greenspan & Benderly, 1997; Renkin, Egeland, Marvinny, Mangelsdorf, & Sroufe, 1989).

Early cognitive experiences are related to the differentiation of emotional responses. Sroufe (1995) suggests that specific emotions evolve with experience from three generalized "state-based" reactions—pleasure/joy, fear, and anger. Early smiles related to physiological sensations become specific, "meaning-based" responses to the occurrence of a pleasurable stimulus, such as the appearance of a familiar person or object, positive social interactions, and mastery/competence experiences. Early fear reactions, such as crying elicited by startling or painful stimuli, develop into more specific "wariness" and then active fear/avoidance responses as the infant learns to distinguish familiar from unfamiliar stimuli and recognize those with "unassimilable" or negative meaning. She begins to be afraid of stimuli she either cannot recognize or recognizes as unpleasant. Early anger reactions, such as "diffuse flailing," are elicited by certain types of physical restraint. These evolve into specific frustration/anger responses when the child is prevented from or unable to carry out intended actions. These reactions strengthen into "rage" during the toddler period. With advancing cognitive development, infants are able to recognize increasing numbers of cues and contexts associated with emotions and begin to experience emotional responses in anticipation or awakened memory of these events.

Both the security of the child's attachments to caregivers and the quality of care provided affect the child's capacity for emotional self-regulation and behavior control (Shore, 1997). Many studies support the importance of early attachment to later social and cognitive development (Gunnar, 1996), and the reliability and responsiveness of the caregiver affects the quality of attachment (Susman-Stillman, Kalkose, Egeland, & Waldman, 1996). Children who receive consistent, responsive care in the first years are more likely to develop positive social skills (Sroufe, 1989).

The development of emotional self-regulation is affected by the quality of the environment, as well the care the child receives (Kopp, 1989; Sroufe, Schork, Motti, Lawroski, & Lafreniere, 1984). Early efforts at self-soothing can be overwhelmed by an overstimulating or chaotic environment or by caregivers who do not notice and support the child's self-regulatory efforts. Early efforts to regulate arousal by engaging with the environment in optimally stimulating ways may be frustrated when the environment does not contain interesting objects and events and people who interact with the child at an age-appropriate level.

The differentiation of emotions, as well as cognitive and motivational development, may be inhibited when the environment does not contain recurrent and predictive cues that can become meaningful to the child. Stimuli that are sometimes positive and sometimes negative, for instance, can generate confusing or ambivalent emotional responses. A predominance of fear- or anger-producing stimuli in the environment can lead to more generally negative emotions and expectations in the child.

EMOTIONAL AND BEHAVIORAL CONTROL IN TODDLE]

The period between 12 and 36 months marks the beginning oi uue voluntary control (12 to 24 months) and the emergence of self-control and self-regulation (24 to 36 months) (Kopp, 1982). There is a qualitative change from the infancy period as children become capable of symbolic representation, language, and self-awareness, which allow the beginnings of "executive" competence and independence. They demonstrate an increasing awareness of their own desires (Erikson, 1963; Nucci et al., 1996), the intentions of others (Meltzoff, 1995), and the requirements of a task (Kopp, 1982, 1992; Rothbart et al., 1992). During the toddler period children begin to be able to form and carry out their own intentions and to comply with external requests to control physical actions, communications, and emotional expression. They are increasingly able to understand and obey external rules and restrictions and to hold themselves back from engaging in prohibited acts. They can also regulate some types of activities by imitating others.

Toddlers are also able to experience more complex emotions, because their understanding is more complex than that of infants. They can not only evaluate and respond to events in context, but can evaluate their own behavior in relation to external standards (what is forbidden and what is allowed) and their own feelings (Sroufe, 1995). With their dawning self-awareness, they begin to experience rudimentary pride in their own capacities and accomplishments and shame at their failures and transgressions. They are pleased when they take off their coats or complete a puzzle successfully and distressed when they engage in a forbidden behavior, especially if caught.

Although their ability to act independently is growing and their desire to do so is growing even faster, toddlers are still very dependent on caregivers. They judge their own behaviors largely by the positive or negative reactions of others and look for cues from them ("social referencing") when they are uncertain. They also frequently need the caregiver's help and support to maintain control in the face of stress, fatigue, or challenge. Adults must set and maintain the standards for behavior, anticipate difficult or frustrating situations, and assist a child who is losing control—while continuing to allow her to be as self-directed as possible (Sroufe, 1995).

Both maturation and experience facilitate the growth of central (executive) control over behavior during the second and third years. Advances in brain development and organization allow the child to inhibit behaviors more effectively and shift more rapidly between emotional states (Schore, 1994). Language also develops rapidly during this period and contributes to both social and cognitive development. Although language plays an important role in the development of self-regulation and control, the external language of caregivers is more effective in producing self-control than the child's own language during the second and third years (Luria, 1961; Vygotsky, 1962). Initially, the child learns to govern her actions according to the rules and requirements of those around her, and these rules are gradually internalized as standards of behavior. During the preschool years the child's own language begins to become a vehicle for self-regulation (Luria, 1961).

As toddlers begin to understand that they are independent beings and have choices, they try to take control of their own activities. They also test their ability to influence or control both objects and other people. They order others about and expect immediate compliance. They are not patient and may have a temper tantrum if crossed. Words like "no" and "mine" are heard frequently. Toddlers' growing understanding of language makes it an increasingly effective means of influencing their behavior, and early self-control appears first as the ability to comply with external requests. However, although toddlers are more able to follow simple directions and to comply with requests or prohibitions, they are also more likely to resist external control.

Kopp (1992) distinguishes between voluntary noncompliance and failure to carry out requests because of incapacity. Sometimes the child is not able to control a behavior or an emotional outburst on demand. Kopp also distinguishes among different types of resistance. Resistance may be demonstrated by "negativism" (kicking, crying, throwing, screaming "no"), "ignoring" a request, "arguing" ("Why do I have to?"), or "off-task negotiation," which involves attempts to distract the caregiver or modify the request (1992, p. 45).

Children between 1 and 3 are not skilled in managing their emotions. Although they show signs of empathy and caring (Eisenberg & Mussen, 1989) and some understanding of the intentions of others (Meltzoff, 1995), they tend to use physical aggression if frustrated or angry. They may also cry or have temper tantrums under these conditions (Kopp, 1992). As difficult and defiant as toddlers may appear, their willfulness signals the possibility of increased internal control. They are trying very hard to take over the management of themselves but are not yet very skilled. They must also learn what is permitted by adults and the society around them (Nucci et al., 1996). It may not be easy for the caregiver to see the power and promise of the 2-year-old's "no," but, if handled appropriately, it contains the seeds of both persistence and self-control. A young child who is too apathetic, confused, or frightened to attempt control may need support in learning to care about and pursue her own goals.

Importance of Experience

The social responsiveness of caregivers and the methods of guidance they use are especially important during these challenging years. Parents and caregivers mediate cultural norms and constraints to children by modeling and verbally transmitting information about what behaviors are acceptable and how much autonomy and control they are permitted (Nucci et al., 1996). Caregiver responses also shape children's sense of self and their expectancies about how others will respond to them. Children's accumulating sets of expectations about their effectiveness in the environment affect their perception of control and willingness to attempt to achieve it.

Many researchers believe that the development of self-control in young children grows out of the quality of the infant–caregiver relationship. They propose that the security generated by early responsive care, and repeated experiences of being able to use an available, trusted caregiver as a base for exploring the environment, lead to a positive and cooperative attitude toward autonomy (Ainsworth & Bell, 1972; Sroufe, 1995). In support of this view, there is evidence that socialization experiences produce neurohormonal changes in the developing brain (Schore, 1994). Sroufe (1995) suggests that different experiences can therefore lead to differences in the brain circuits that mediate emotions and result in "variations in the autoregulation of affect and self-regulation more generally" (p. 203).

Through the process of socialization, children come to internalize the values and behavior expectations of the family and the culture. Internalization is the process through which external rules become internal standards that guide self-regulated behavior (Ryan & Stiller, 1991). Compliance is distinguished from internalization because it is a response to external control (Lepper, 1983). The goal of socialization is to have the child internalize values and standards, which she will then use to guide her own behavior in a variety of settings without the need for constant external supervision and control. As socialization proceeds, caregivers can begin to shift control to the child in age- and skill-appropriate areas.

Research suggests that the process of internalization is more effectively supported by certain types of guidance strategies and styles. The conditions that promote compliance and caregiver control over the child's behavior may not be the same as those that promote subsequent internalization of values and standards. Coercive control, which gains compliance by means of external rewards, punishments, or physical force, undermines the processes that lead to internal control (Lepper, 1983). Strategies that emphasize individual control over behavior (Lepper, 1981), use suggestions rather than commands (Lepper, 1981; Maccoby, 1980), and focus on explanations and reasoning rather than power-assertive demands for compliance (Hoffman, 1970b) are most likely to support the development of internal control.

Parental demands and styles of control also influence the development of self-regulated social competence (Kuzynski & Kochanska, 1995; Rothbaum & Crockenberg, 1995). A number of recent studies suggest that a "collaborative" approach, in which the goals of both children and parents are considered, is effective in promoting social skills (Crockenberg et al., 1996). Using problem-solving techniques, solutions are negotiated that take into account the concerns of all parties. With very young children this "negotiation" requires caregivers to take the child's interest in self-direction into account by providing appropriate opportunities for choice. The older, more verbal child, with a greater appreciation of the perspectives of others, can learn to negotiate more actively and independently.

EMOTIONAL AND BEHAVIORAL CONTROL IN PRESCHOOL AND KINDERGARTEN CHILDREN

In contrast to toddlers, who typically need guidance and support from adults in their self-regulatory activities, preschool and kindergarten children are increasingly capable of true internal self-regulation that uses rules, strategies, and plans to guide behavior (Kopp, 1982). They are also beginning to use speech as a technique for controlling both action and thought (Berk & Winsler, 1995; Fuson, 1979; Luria, 1961; Vygotsky, 1962; Zivin, 1979). Children in this age range are more able to control their behavior, and the way they express emotions in interactions with other people, than younger children (Achenbach & Edelbrock, 1981, 1991; Eisenberg & Fabes, 1992; Eisenberg, Fabes, & Losoya, 1997; Eisenberg, Fabes, Shepard, et al., 1997). They are interested in spending more time with other children and need to become more skilled in managing their emotions and behaviors in order to interact with and influence others successfully (Bronson, 1994; Dodge, 1985; Dodge, Pettit, McClasky, & Brown, 1986; Howes, 1988; Ladd, Price, & Hart, 1990; Parten, 1932).

During the preschool and kindergarten period children are increasingly *expected* to be able to regulate their emotions and behaviors appropriately. Their goals become clearer and more conscious, but they are expected to be able to "delay, defer, and accept substitutions without becoming aggressive or disorganized by frustration, and . . . cope well with high arousal, whether due to environmental challenge or fatigue" (Sroufe, 1995, p. 214). Their increased symbolic and representational capacities may help children in this age range express emotions in play, and psychoanalytic theory suggests that they can "work through" difficult or painful feelings in fantasy play (Breger, 1973). Sroufe, Cooper, and De Hart (1996) suggested that fantasy play is a major tool for emotional self-regulation during this period.

Another major tool for emotional and behavioral self-regulation during this period is language, which becomes an increasingly important mediator of self-regulation in action and thought from the preschool period onward. Bronowski (1977) suggested several properties of language that assist in maintaining control. As an aid to memory, language helps the individual refer backward in time and project forward into the future, allowing more adequate learning from past experience and planning for the future. Language assists emotional regulation by permitting a separation between the emotional and factual content of a communication or message. Language assists internal thought, reflection, and planning by facilitating the child's mental consideration of alternatives before acting. It also facilitates the construction, reconstruction, and recombination of material in memory to form new concepts, plans, and solutions to problems.

Vygotsky (1962) suggested that self-speech (thinking and giving oneself directions in words) begins during the preschool years and is critical for the development of self-regulated behavior. Overt self-speech typically increases until about age 7 (Fuson, 1979), when it declines and becomes internalized in silent thought (or "subvocal speech") (Vygotsky, 1962). As children grow older they gradually become able to use self-speech to consciously understand situations, focus on problems, and overcome difficulties (Harris, 1990; Zivin, 1979). Bickhard (1990) suggests that children (and adults) can use verbal supports for ongoing activities ("self-scaffolding") in both task and social situations and proposes that self-scaffolding is central and essential for cognitive control. The young child's speech during tasks or fantasy play can often reveal the presence of self-organizing and self-regulating strategies (Bronson, 1985; Berk, 1994; Goodwin, 1981).

Preschool and kindergarten children require less continuous adult support and guidance to maintain appropriate behavior. They are now more able and more likely to comply with the rules of behavior adults provide, and to carry out age-appropriate requests and directions in both home and school settings. They can use adults as resources for learning or assistance when necessary but are less dependent on their intervention and constant monitoring than younger children. During this period children internalize standards for behavior and begin to monitor their own actions (Kopp, 1982). There is a gradual shift from external to internal control.

Adults are still central to the lives of preschool and kindergarten children, but, from ages 3 through 5, peers become increasingly important to them. Success in establishing relationships with peers is a central issue in development during this period. The ability to regulate emotions and control behavior becomes increasingly necessary for age-appropriate interactions with others (Eisenberg & Fabes, 1992; Eisenberg et al., 1993), and an attitude of negotiation and reciprocity replaces the toddler's insistence on having her own way.

Importance of Experience

The ability to engage in self-directed and rewarding interactions with peers grows dramatically during this period, and competence in peer relations is extremely important from these ages onward. Social competence in the preschool and kindergarten years requires emotion regulation, social knowledge and understanding, and specific social skills (Katz & McClellan, 1997). Emotion regulation and the ability to use specific social skills or strategies effectively require inhibition of inappropriate behaviors and positive self-directed approaches to others. These competencies, as well as advances in social knowledge and understanding, require practice and guidance in interaction with other people (Asher & Renshaw, 1981; Mize & Ladd, 1990).

The development of self-regulated social competence is supported by interactions with both adults and peers. Adults provide models and verbal guidelines for social and emotional actions and attitudes. They have a great influence on children's social interest and involvement, on their social interaction patterns and styles, and on their social understanding. Relations between children and their primary caregivers provide models and expectations for social exchange (Rudolph, Harmen, & Burge, 1995). The child's attachment to the caregiver (Ainsworth & Bell, 1974) and the caregiver's loving interest in the child (Bronfenbrenner, 1990) influence the child's developing sense of self and her interactions with others. The trust, security, warmth, and caring experienced in early relationships influence children's later relationships with the social and material world. Relatedness to others provides a social context that supports internalization of the rules and values in the child's world (Goodenow, 1993; Ryan & Powelson, 1991).

The caregiver's guidance methods also influence self-control and social competence. "Authoritative," rather than permissive or authoritarian, control supports the child's internalization of social guidelines (Baumrind, 1967, 1973). A balance of warmth and firm guidance that is appropriate to the child's age and understanding and supports developing inner control, leads to both independence and sociability (Baumrind, 1967). As with younger children, a collaborative approach, which considers the goals of all parties concerned, supports the development of inner control (Crockenberg et al., 1996) and coercive control undermines it (Lepper, 1981). Interactions between socially competent preschool children and their mothers are marked by coherence, reciprocity, and contingency of the mothers' responses to their children's behavior (Dumas & LaFreniere, 1993).

Parents' guidance styles also influence the prevalence of negative behaviors (Russell & Russell, 1996), children's ability to engage in social problem solving (Rose-Krasnor, Rubin, Booth, & Coplan, 1996), and overall social competence (Kuczynski & Kochanska, 1995; Rothbaum & Crockenberg, 1995). Emotional competence and the incidence of positive social behaviors can also be increased by caregiver modeling and scaffolding (Denham, Mason, & Couchoud, 1995; Denham, Mitchell-Copeland, Strandberg, Blair, & Auerbach, 1997; Eisenberg & Mussen, 1989). Caregiver attitudes and behaviors have important effects on children's self-regulation and social competence.

Peers also have an important role in the development of social control and competence (Dunn, 1996; Hartup, 1983; Parker & Asher, 1987). Children who participate in social interactions with peers develop more advanced cognitive, linguistic, and social skills (Doise, 1990; Guralnick, 1981; Parker & Gottman, 1989; Rubin & Pepler, 1980) and develop effective strategies for communicating (Garvey, 1986; Shure, 1981; Strayer, 1989). Too much peer dependence in young children may be a cause for concern, because adults are better sources of guidance for children than peers (Katz & McClellan, 1997). However, if children have little access to peers or are rejected by them, important sources of learning are lost.

The negative effects of social rejection are well documented (Achenbach & Edelbrock, 1981, 1991; Asher & Wheeler, 1985; Dodge et al., 1986; Howes, 1988). Long-term consequences associated with lack of competent social interaction with peers include delinquency, school failure, and various forms of psychopathology (Kupersmidt, Coie, & Dodge, 1990; Parker & Asher, 1987; Rubin, Chen, & Hymel, 1993). In addition, a variety of studies have shown that many indicators of social competence and social rejection are relatively stable from early to middle childhood (Asendorpf, 1989; Dodge, 1983; Howes, 1990; Ladd et al., 1990; Putallaz, 1983). Other longitudinal research has confirmed the long-term significance of specific social and emotional variables. Peer interaction skills, peer acceptance, motivation, and self-concept have been correlated with higher levels of functioning in school and in life (Berrueta-Clement, Schweinhart, Barnett, Epstein, & Weikart, 1984; Bronson, Pierson, & Tivnan, 1984; Hauser-Cram, Pierson, Walker, & Tivnan, 1991; Kemple, 1991; Ladd & Price, 1989; Lazare & Darlington, 1982; Pellegrini, 1992). The implications are that a lack of peer interaction skills and peer acceptance may be related to difficulties in establishing peer relationships in the middle childhood years, which in turn appear to predict adjustment in adulthood (Odom, McConnell, & McEvoy, 1992).

Adult support for constructive peer relationships and modes of interaction is important because the effects of peer neglect are so enduring (Coie & Dodge, 1983; Parker & Asher, 1987; Putallaz & Gottman, 1981). Inadequate, unsuccessful, or aggressive patterns of interaction may continue into elementary school and later life. Mere exposure to other children is not enough to create social competence (Clarke-Stewart, Gruber, & Fitzgerald, 1994). Although preschool and kindergarten children's capacity for internal control is growing they still sometimes need individualized guidance from adults to support impulse control and social problem solving and to strengthen prosocial dispositions. Children may also need adult help to accommodate to individual differences, other children's wishes and suggestions, and frustration when things do not go well (Katz & McClellan, 1997).

EMOTIONAL AND BEHAVIORAL CONTROL
IN PRIMARY SCHOOL CHILDREN

Parents and teachers agree that self-regulation in the social area is important. They rate social skills, goal-directedness, and emotional stability as more likely to lead to school and life success than variables such as IQ and aptitude (Getzels & Jackson, 1963). Many preschool and elementary school programs stress the development of interpersonal skills and the ability to get along cooperatively with others, and teachers' reports of social and emotional status have been used as a basis for placement decisions (Bowman & Svetina, 1992). Elementary school teachers emphasize social competence as well as cognitive achievements in their evaluations of children (Fry, 1984). They value positive and cooperative behavior (Pallas, Entwisle, Alexander, & Cadigan, 1987), the appropriate regulation of emotions (Alexander & Entwisle, 1988), and following classroom rules and adult requests (McKim & Cowen, 1987; Reynolds, 1991).

In a series of large longitudinal studies of children's performance over the first few grades in school, teachers' ratings of children's "conduct" were highly predictive of later reading and academic performance (Entwisle, Alexander, Cadigan, & Pallas, 1986; Entwisle & Hayduk, 1982). These studies suggest that, in addition to the fact that children with social problems experience many long-term difficulties, those who exhibit more disruptive behavior may be less successfully engaged in the educational aspects of the classroom as well. Children who participate actively and positively in the educational aspects of school demonstrate subsequent successful school achievement (Finn & Cox, 1992).

Self-regulation of emotion and behavior is not only important for a judgment of adequacy by adults. Peer rejection of children in this age range is associated with both "externalizing disorders," such as aggression, inappropriate behavior or hyperactivity, and "internalizing disorders," such as negative emotionality or withdrawn behaviors (Dodge, 1983; Eisenberg et al., 1996). Research has linked both of these types of disorder to problems in regulating emotion (Eisenberg et al., 1996), and both are related to social difficulties in later childhood and adolescence (Dodge, 1983; Rubin, Hymel, & Mills, 1989).

Most of the self-regulating or "executive" functions are well under way in development by the early school years, but are not fully internalized until early adolescence (Barkley, 1997). There is a noticeable increase in self-regulation in the 5-to-7 age range (Berkowitz, 1982), and shifts in mental functioning during this period have been noted by psychologists as diverse as Freud (1920), Erikson (1963), Piaget (1970), and Sheldon White (1970). Children become more responsible and more consciously aware of themselves, their actions and thoughts. The development of self-regulation can now be assisted not only by supporting the development and exercise of self-regulatory skills, but by supporting children's conscious awareness and conscious use of such skills (Donaldson, 1978, 1987).

A variety of explanations have been suggested for the improvement in the regulation of emotions and behavior during this period. Some focus on the internalization of language and its use as a support for self-regulation. Some stress the importance of increased control of attention. Other explanations focus on the increased cognitive and information-processing capacities of children in this age range and the accompanying improvements in their ability to distinguish emotional responses, understand the requirements of different situations, and mobilize appropriate coping strategies.

Vygotsky (1962) and Luria (1961) suggested the importance of self-speech, which becomes internalized during these years (Berk, 1992), for self-regulation. They thought that the ability to use internalized language to identify internal states and external conditions, and to plan and direct behavioral responses, is basic to all forms of self-regulation. Others have noted that language can (1) increase the distinctiveness of certain stimulus attributes of a situation, (2) direct the child's attention to the relevant dimensions of a problem, (3) assist the child in forming hypotheses and plans about how to proceed with a task, and (4) help the child maintain the relevant dimensions in short-term memory (Meichenbaum, 1977).

The ability to control attention has also been related to effective regulation of emotion and behavior (Eisenberg et al., 1996; Mischel, 1974; Skinner, 1948). The ability to divert attention from an over-arousing or unpleasant stimulus and focus on positive aspects of the situation, or on strategies for coping, is associated with more effective regulation of emotion and control of behavior. Attention control has been related to lower levels of negative emotions, such as distress and frustration, and higher levels of peer popularity, appropriate social behavior, and constructive management of anger (Eisenberg, Fabes, et al., 1997).

Emotion regulation requires a number of cognitive skills (Kopp, 1989), and early elementary school children have an expanded capacity for cognitive processing in comparison with younger children. Piaget (1970) describes their emergence from "egocentrism" and increased ability to take the perspective of others. Using an information-processing model, Garber et al. (1991) suggest that competent emotion regulation requires a number of specific cognitive steps, which older children are better able to accomplish. These include (1) *perception* that affect is aroused and needs to be regulated, (2) *interpretation* of what is causing the arousal and who is responsible for doing something about it, (3) *goal setting*, a decision about what needs to be done, (4) *generation of responses* to reach the goal, (5) *evaluation* of the probable outcome in terms of both the goal and one's own competence, and (6) *performance* of the selected responses. They propose that this model provides a framework for describing and evaluating competent versus "maladjusted" emotional regulation.

Researchers have distinguished between behavioral (external) and cognitive (internal) strategies to regulate emotions and between "emotion-focused" and "problem-focused" strategies, which can also be viewed as external (emotion focused) or internal (problem focused) (Brenner & Salovey, 1997). The use of internal strategies increases with development. In addition, children's overall store of regulatory strategies increases with age and experience and they become better at distinguishing between controllable and uncontrollable situations. Mischel and Mischel (1983) suggest that the child's conscious knowledge of self-control strategies begins during the early elementary years and becomes increasingly sophisticated.

In summary, early elementary school children are able to control emotional expression and behavior more effectively than younger children. They have better control of attention and can use internalized language for self-regulation. They become more self-aware and begin to be able to reflect consciously and make deliberate decisions about courses of action in different situations. They are also beginning to understand the feelings and perspectives of others more clearly and are able to work and play with them more cooperatively. An increased understanding of the feelings and perspectives of others allows them to more consciously adjust their own emotions and behaviors to the emotions and behaviors of others. As they become more proficient in making these adjustments they are able to engage not only in more complex personal interactions with others, but in joint work projects and relatively independent "cooperative learning" activities with other children.

Importance of Experience

The cumulative effects of early social experiences affect the child's emotional and behavioral control in elementary school. Many experiences with others have been transformed into internalized models for self-guidance or "generalized cognitive representations of relationships" (Rudolph et al., 1995, p. 1393), which affect both the way the child behaves and the way she interprets the behaviors of others. Social learning theorists suggest that through cumulative direct and vicarious (observing others) experiences, individuals develop "performance standards" in a number of areas, which they use to guide (self-regulate) and evaluate their own behavior (Bandura, 1977, 1997). They cognitively reward or punish themselves according to their perceived ability to live up to these internalized standards and experience feelings of competence or self-efficacy when they are able to meet them. Performance standards become more clearly discriminated and realistic with age and experience. A self-conscious 7-year-old may experience anguish over her failure to read as well as others in the class, whereas a 4-year-old may exclaim proudly that she can "read" when she is able to look through a book and remember some words of the story. Early elementary school children are beginning to evaluate themselves more clearly and consciously in relation to others and are particularly vulnerable to external negative judgments and comparisons.

Experiences with parents are important because of their continuity with the past and because the parent–child relationship is exposed to new challenges during the early elementary years. Sroufe (1995) notes:

> Not only are the parents' stated values and those behaviors that are praised and proscribed, but the practiced patterns of dyadic regulation are internalized by the child . . . [and] such internalization is both physiological and cognitive, influencing basic orientations (expectations) and affective responses to interpersonal situations, as well as more conscious beliefs and values, and influencing attitudes as well as behavioral style. (p. 232)

He argued for a "coherence over time" in which "early patterns of caregiver-guided regulation predict to dyadic regulation (attachment patterns) and to later parental acceptance of autonomy and promotion of instrumentality" (pp. 228–229). As the child develops, the "connectedness" is not dissolved but is "transformed" as parents support the child's growing independence, allowing as much self-regulated activity as she is capable of at each age. Early close and secure relationships provide the basis for children's ability to engage in autonomous self-regulated activities.

Researchers have also found relationships between problem behaviors in school-age children and parental problems. Research by
Cummings and colleagues (Cummings, Hennessy, & Sugarman,
1984; Cummings, Simpson, & Wilson, 1993; Cummings, Zahn-
Waxler, & Radke-Yarrow, 1994) shows the negative effects of exposure to parental anger on children. Children exposed to repeated
angry parental conflicts tended to cope with conflict by using maladaptive strategies such as physical aggression, and children whose
mothers had high scores on an anger measure were more likely to express anger when provoked than those whose mothers scored low on
this measure. Parents in aggressive families are more likely to label
neutral events as antisocial (Patterson, 1986), so children from these
environments may have more situations to perceive as warranting
negative reactions. Parental depression, as well, appears to affect
children's self-regulatory abilities (Dix, 1991; Downey & Coyne,
1990; Garber et al., 1991). Depressed mothers tend to be more critical, hostile, and negative and less emotionally expressive and cooperative with their children, and the children appear to model these
strategies in their interactions with others. Brenner and Salovey
(1997) note that parents actively teach their children how to regulate
emotion and that children's observed behaviors, both positive and
negative, reflect this teaching. For instance, parents who encourage
their children to express emotion in socially appropriate ways are
more likely to have empathetic, emotionally expressive children
(Eisenberg et al., 1991; Eisenberg & Fabes, 1992).

Experiences with peers are increasingly important for elementary school children. From the preschool period onward, the peer
group becomes a source of learning about emotional self-regulation
(Barkley, 1997). Social problems during preschool, especially those
resulting from a lack of appropriate control of emotions or behavior, or a lack of positive skills for approaching and interacting with
peers, tend to follow the child into elementary school and beyond
(Coie & Dodge, 1983; Parker & Asher, 1987; Putallaz & Gottman, 1981).

During the early elementary school period children become more
consciously aware of themselves in relation to their peers and more
vulnerable to peer judgments. They are eager to be accepted by their
peers, and rejected children are vulnerable to later adjustment problems (Asher & Dodge, 1986). Children in this age range are also be-

coming increasingly involved in *peer-regulated* activities, and their emotional and behavioral expression in these situations is somewhat influenced by the norms of the group.

As peer influences become stronger, they may begin to challenge the influence of the family. Some research suggests that children who are independent from their parents but have positive and close relationships with them, and come from homes that provide high levels of nurturance and support with firm but not oppressive discipline, are less vulnerable to negative peer influences (Kandel & Lesser, 1972). The parents of extremely peer-oriented children exhibit both less support and less control of their children and demonstrate lower levels of concern and affection for them (Condry & Siman, 1974). Gang-orientation has been associated with either a high level of permissiveness or a high level of punitiveness in the home (Devereux, 1970).

The larger environment increasingly influences young school-age children's emotional and behavioral self-regulation. They may, for example, be exposed to a wider range of television programs, and their viewing may be less supervised by adults and less subject to critical evaluation. The effects of negative exposure in this case is clear: the relationship between media violence and aggressive behaviors in children is well documented (Parke & Slaby, 1983). As children reach out to the world beyond the family, media and peer and other nonfamily models become particularly salient.

SUMMARY

The development of appropriate emotional and behavioral control is extremely important. Self-regulation in these areas is related to social competence, to acceptance by peers, to school success, and to life adjustment. Although there are some genetic tendencies such as temperament that influence development, the environment—and particularly the social environment—exerts powerful shaping influences.

The child comes equipped with a few innate mechanisms for controlling arousal and emotional expression, but soon begins to develop more specific and effective strategies. The development of control has been explained in different ways by different theories, but all agree that there is a general movement from mediated or assisted control to more independent self-regulation, which is affected by both maturation and experience. The caregiver appears to be particularly important in the establishment of early patterns of control, and early patterns affect future development.

The development of control is inseparable from overall social and cognitive development. Cognitive interpretation and affect are linked to create "meaning" and discriminated emotional and behavioral responses. Caregivers provide the sense of security, personal acceptance, and "trust" in the environment that many believe are essential for positive emotional development. The larger social environment provides social rules, models, and consequences (rewards and punishments) that shape the child's goals and behavioral expressions.

Control over emotions and behavior changes with age and experience. During the first 3 months of life, infants begin to adapt their innate regulatory systems to the environment and develop internal control mechanisms that allow some self-directed voluntary control of arousal. In the period between 3 and 12 months babies expand their repertoire of responses and begin to initiate interactions with people and objects. By the end of this period they can begin to respond to simple one-step external commands.

During the first year, the role of caregivers is particularly important for the child's development. Caregivers help set daily rhythms and regulate arousal during the first 3 months. Regular and responsive care allows the child to begin to feel secure and begin to develop organized patterns of responses. Throughout the first year, interactions with others help the child to discriminate between the self and others and begin to develop voluntary control strategies. These interactions also facilitate the development of close and secure attachments to primary caregivers, which many theorists believe support healthy emotional development and the gradual growth of autonomy.

The toddler period marks the beginning of true voluntary control (12 to 24 months) and the emergence of self-control (24 to 36 months). Children become capable of symbolic representation and language and develop a beginning awareness of their own desires, the intentions of others, and the requirements of a task. They are beginning to understand external constraints but are more interested in exercising control, especially over their own behavior. Because toddlers' interest in regulating their own activities is not matched by their ability to control either behavior or emotions, this period can be stressful for both children and caregivers.

Adult guidance and support are especially important during these years. A combination of firm but responsive guidance and support for the child's autonomy and attempts at self control is most likely to foster cooperation and increased self-regulation. Respect for the child's growing need for independence and a "collaborative" attitude help the child develop inner controls. Power-assertive demands for compliance invite resistance and foster reactive attempts to control in the child.

Preschool and kindergarten children are increasingly capable of true internal self-regulation that uses internalized rules, strategies, and plans to guide behavior. Their increased symbolic capacities help them express and work through their feelings in play. They are also beginning to use language to help them understand emotions and problem situations and to negotiate and resolve problems. Children in this age range are also more able and eager to comply with adult requests. As they internalize standards for behavior and emotional expression, there is a gradual shift from external to internal control.

Preschool and kindergarten children need less adult supervision than toddlers, but they still need adults to plan the environment to support their efforts at self-regulation and to step in when control fails. A child's attachment to primary caregivers and the caregivers' loving interest in the child continue to support her sense of self and her autonomous control. As with toddlers, so too with preschool and kindergarten children, parenting styles that are consistent but responsive to the child's needs, and supportive of growing independence, contribute to the development of emotional and behavioral self-regulation. A lack of external guidelines or the use of coercive control undermines the development of self-control. In addition, parents' own interpersonal strategies and styles of interaction provide models that children internalize and imitate.

Peers also become important during the preschool and kindergarten years. Their behavior provides models, and their responses provide feedback to the child about her own competence. The types of interactions with peers the child experiences help shape her own behavior and expectations in the future.

Primary school children have an increased ability to control emotions and behavior. They have better control of attention and can use internalized language to guide behavior. They are better able to understand the perspectives of others and can better understand their own and others' wishes and feelings. Their information-processing capacities, including memory, are improved, and they have an increased number of control strategies at their command. They are also more self-aware and can begin to reflect on their own actions and feelings. They are beginning to compare themselves with others and their behavior with internalized performance standards. This means that sense of self is greatly expanded but they are also more vulnerable to negative feedback.

Experiences with parents are still important during this period. The child's cumulative experience with caregivers and the continuing support she receives is a major support for development, but the child's world is becoming larger. She is becoming more actively involved and committed to the models and opinions provided by peers and other influences outside the home. She is more aware of this larger world and is beginning to consciously test her skills and her ability to meet and master the challenges it presents.

Table 3.1 summarizes the development of emotional and behavioral control in the four age ranges and the major effects of the environment at each age.

TABLE 3.1. The Development of Emotional and Behavioral Control and Effects of the Environment on This Development

Development of emotional and behavioral control	Effects of the environment
Infants	
Develop self-soothing and self-stimulating strategies	Chaotic, overstimulating, or understimulating environment impedes development of adaptive arousal and wake–sleep patterns
Develop arousal and sleep–wake patterns that relate to the environment	
Begin voluntary efforts to control own motor activity and behaviors	Caregiver warmth and responsiveness assists development of differentiated emotional responses
Begin voluntary efforts to contact other people and objects and to engage in sustained interactions with them	Caregiver warmth, consistency, and responsiveness to child's signals support feelings of security and development of awareness of control
	Caregiver responsive interactions with infant establishes early understanding of social interaction and communication patterns (turn-taking, etc.)
Toddlers	
Experience more complex emotions	Caregiver sensitivity to child's needs and individual characteristics supports the development of inner control
Develop early impulse control (can comply with simple directions and restrictions)	
Develop language and increasing awareness of own desires (can form and carry out intentions)	Environments arranged for safe independent action and self-testing, with opportunities for positive experiences with objects and peers, support the development of inner control
Can regulate some types of activities by imitating others	Positive models of behavior support the development of self-regulated control
Use social referencing to judge own actions and environmental events	Positive and responsive guidance that is consistent but respects autonomy and encourages responsibility and self-control supports self-regulation
Prekindergarten and kindergarten	
Increasingly capable of true internal control of emotions and behavior	Caregiver guidance techniques and styles that support responsibility, inner control, and positive interactions with others support the development of self-regulation
Need less continuous adult support and guidance to maintain control (shifting from external to internal control)	
More interest in interacting with other children and being accepted by them	Adult and peer modeling influence children's patterns of interaction, self-control, and developing standards for appropriate behavior
Capable of cooperative interactions with peers	Opportunities for positive interactions with peers that include adult monitoring of peer interactions, mediating disputes (if necessary) in a problem-solving way, and an expressed value for cooperative interactions, increase positive self-regulation
Able to use internalized rules, strategies, and plans to guide behavior (though not necessarily consciously)	
Internalizing standards for appropriate behavior and emotional expression	
Can use language to assist and guide self-regulation	
Primary school	
Major shift between ages 5 and 7 in responsibility and internal self-regulation	Cumulative effects of early experience (first 5 years) affects both behavior and standards of performance (how the child believes she "should" act and how she evaluates her own behavior)
Capable of reliable internal regulation of behavior and emotional expression	
Can follow and stick to rules	Rules, standards of behavior, and observed behaviors of others in the current environment continue to influence the child's developing internal standards, values, and expressed behaviors
Able to use self-speech to regulate thoughts and actions	
Can usually negotiate disputes with peers independently	Family interaction patterns and the family climate of communication continue to influence developing self-regulation, but peer (and media) influences and standards are increasingly powerful
Consciously aware of self and capacity for self-regulation	
Consciously aware of and more able to understand the feelings and perspectives of others	Guidance strategies that support internal control and responsibility continue to be important in supporting internal self-regulation
Judge own behavior and behavior of others according to internalized standards of behavior (but these are often rigid and punitive)	
Interested in "fairness"	

4

Engaging in Prosocial Behavior

The general public is interested not only in the exercise of self-control but in what types of behaviors individual control produces. Political and ethical leaders, the popular press, parents, and teachers are interested in self-regulation that leads *toward* positive social activities and *away from* antisocial behaviors. They want to know how to promote social responsibility and decrease violence and crime.

Positive social behaviors have typically been called "prosocial," moral, or altruistic by psychologists. There has been some difficulty in providing general definitions for these positive activities because the particular behaviors considered prosocial in one setting or group may not be the same, or even equivalent, in different settings or groups. For instance, physical force and hostile aggression may be considered acceptable or desirable in very few situations by some groups, and in very many situations by others.

The definition difficulty applies not only to different cultural groups but also to different ages, genders, settings, and social groups within the same cultural group. Two-year-olds are not expected to perform the same helping, sharing, or comforting activities expected of 12-year-olds, and a dangerous situation that would appropriately send a 2-year-old running to an adult might require the adult or an older child to protect and defend the toddler. Aggression might be more acceptable (or encouraged) in boys than in girls, while girls might be expected to be more empathetic or nurturing. Expectations for behavior toward family, friends, or members of a club might differ from expectations for behavior toward those outside these groups.

In order to understand increases in the tendency to engage in positive social behaviors in young children and how this growth can be supported, it is necessary to review the ways prosocial development has been described and explained in the psychological literature. This literature includes both theory and research on the development of prosocial and altruistic behavior and moral understanding. Theoretical perspectives differ in interesting and important ways, providing a variety of explanations for the development of prosocial behaviors and dispositions. The research literature documents (1) the kinds of behaviors considered positive or prosocial in children, (2) at what ages they have been observed to appear, and (3) the circumstances associated with (and appearing to support) their development.

This chapter begins with an overview of the major theoretical perspectives on prosocial development, focusing on their relation to the development of self-regulation. Following this overview, summaries of the research evidence related to the development of self-regulated prosocial behavior at different early childhood ages are presented. To distinguish and highlight circumstances associated with the appearance of positive behaviors, factors associated with the development of negative behavior patterns are sometimes described as well.

THEORETICAL PERSPECTIVES ON THE DEVELOPMENT OF PROSOCIAL BEHAVIOR

Explanations for the tendency to engage in prosocial or antisocial behaviors have come from ethologists as well as from psychologists. Explanations provided by psychologists have differed from the ethological perspective and from each other. They differ on the source of the tendency to engage in prosocial or antisocial behavior, the types of environmental circumstances that support the development of these tendencies, and the degree to which the behaviors can be considered self-regulated.

The Ethological Perspective

Building on animal models, ethologists have looked for the roots of both prosocial behaviors and aggression in instinctual impulses built into the genes by evolution (Eibl-Eibesfeldt, 1970; Lorenz, 1965, 1966; Wilson, 1975). Lorenz believed that there are four types of instinctual impulses—hunger, sexuality, flight, and aggression—and that even "love," defined as the personal bond, evolved from aggression. Eibl-Eibesfeldt (1970) agrees that aggression is older than individualized social bonds, but proposes that social bonding evolved from the (nonaggressive) parent–child bond. He describes the tendency among primates to use symbolic "threats at a distance" rather than physical aggression to maintain control or dominance over others, especially within their own social groups. He also notes that primates as a whole have peaceful habits and that violent aggression rarely occurs in their natural habitats except under situations of stress and overcrowding.

Wilson (1975) proposes that the nuclear family is the basic building block of all human societies and that the "moralistic rules" underlying social functioning are based on elaborated kinship systems similar in some ways to those operating in hunter-gatherer societies. He notes that "sharing" is rare among nonhuman primates, but that it is one of the strongest human traits. He further suggests that controlled sharing is the basis of human economic systems, which are, in turn, based on extensions of kinship rules. These kinship systems "bind alliances between tribes and subtribal units," provide for the "conflict-free emigration of young members, . . . are an important part of the bartering system by which certain males achieve dominance and leadership," and serve (through sharing) as a "device for seeing groups through hard times" (p. 554).

Wilson also emphasizes the variation among specific rules of social organization and behavior (including sharing) and the cultural relativity of what is considered "ethical" or good. He suggests that although the development of kinship-based systems and rules that promote survival are universal, the content of these systems and rules varies considerably. From the ethological perspective, both aggressive and altruistic tendencies, such as putting the needs of the young or the social group above one's own, are present in humans today because they have contributed to human survival in the past and are now "in the genes."

The Psychoanalytic Perspective

Freud's (1930) theory also assumed an instinctual base for behavior. He proposed that humans have both a life instinct and a death instinct that influence behavior in opposite directions. The life instinct supports engagement in positive, life-affirming activities by contributing energy to constructive work and loving relationships with others. Aggression comes from the death instinct, described as an innate tendency to destroy. Energy derived from this source is usually directed against other people or property, but is sometimes directed against the self whereby it can result in self-destructive actions and even suicide.

Freud (1920, 1965) also suggested a specific internal mechanism, the superego, to account for self-regulated moral behavior. He proposed that the superego develops as the child internalizes the pattern of rewards and punishments she receives. This is largely accomplished by the time the child enters primary school, so early experience is critical. The superego contains both the "conscience" and the "ego ideal." The conscience contains internalized experiences of punishment, which make the child feel guilty when engaging in behaviors that have been punished in the past. The ego ideal contains internalized experiences that have been rewarded. It makes the child feel proud when engaging in, or even thinking about engaging in, previously rewarded behaviors and can act as a source of motivation for positive behaviors. The superego drives (by means of the conscience, which produces guilt) or inspires (by means of the ego ideal) individuals to engage in behaviors that are approved by society (Breger, 1973).

The content and strength of the constraints imposed by the superego are determined both by the child's own biological drives and by the types of sanctions and rewards imposed by the environment. In Freud's formulation the superego constantly strives for perfection and is as unrealistic in its demands as the instinctual drives of the id. The individual's mental life is often in conflict as the rational ego tries to mediate between the opposing demands of the id and the superego. The goal of the ego is to produce reasonable gratification for the id that does not offend the superego. It guides the individual to engage in prosocial or altruistic behaviors only when this gratifies the superego and does not violate the demands of the id.

Later theorists in the psychoanalytic tradition are less pessimistic about human nature and view self-regulation as freer from conflict. They see the individual as less isolated from others (Adler, 1956; Erikson, 1963), individual goals as less opposed to the requirements of society (Adler, 1956; Erikson, 1959), and development as less constrained by the effects of early experience (Horney, 1945; Erikson, 1963). They also propose that the ego has energy and goals of its own, thus freeing this self-regulatory function from domination by the id, and the superego and from its warring role with society (Erikson, 1963; White, 1963; May, 1967). Proposed ego goals include competence (White, 1963), self-fulfillment (Maslow, 1968, 1970; May, 1953; Rogers, 1963), and the development of meaning and values (May, 1967). May (1969) describes a love for others that goes beyond sex (*eros*), and even friendship (*philia*), to unselfish concern for the welfare of others (*agape*). This love is unconditional, like the love of a parent or the "love of God for man" (p. 319). Self-regulated behavior motivated by agape is both prosocial and altruistic.

The Behavioral Perspective

Behavioral theorists have proposed that learned habits and conditioned associations between certain social behaviors and rewards, combined with conditioned negative associations between other behaviors and punishments, can account for both "conscience" and prosocial behavior patterns (Eysenck, 1960, 1976). They generally emphasize the role of the environment in shaping positive and negative behaviors, but some connections between aggression and genetic tendencies have been suggested. Aggression has not been considered a biological drive like the need for food or sex; however, an innate link with frustration was proposed by early social learning theorists (Dollard, Doob, Miller, Mowrer, & Sears, 1939).

More recent analyses have classified aggression as either "impulsive" (uncontrolled) attempts to reach goals (one child grabbing a toy from another or hitting a child who has taken her toy) or self-regulated (controlled) aggression deliberately employed as a means to reach a goal (Logue, 1995). The child gradually develops the ability to control impulsive behavior and wait for delayed rewards in order to reach desired goals. Self-control is considered "proactive behavior—either overt or covert—that we do at one time to control our later behaviors" (Baldwin & Baldwin, 1998, p. 352). It consists of "behavioral chains" that include at least five basic components: self-observation, self-description, self-evaluation (in terms of valued goals), self-instruction, and reinforcement (which can include external or internal self-reinforcement).

Behavioral theory does not specify types of prosocial behaviors (such as sharing or helping) or goals (such as producing benefits for others), because these are viewed as environmentally determined. Particular behaviors are strategies for reaching desired goals, and the benefits of specific behaviors or goals are considered in relation to the satisfaction of the individual. Both goals and the self-control skills required to reach them are learned. The environment provides models, rules, prompts (helpful verbal or other cues), and reinforcement for learning, and learning begins when children are very young. Parents and peers, as well as other salient people and events in the child's life, determine the content of this learning.

Behavioral learning theorists have focused on how the external environment shapes children's ability to exercise internal control over behavior (Logue, 1995). They assume that the environment teaches children to select appropriate (socially approved) rewards and to wait for appropriate (socially approved) times and places to receive them. Children learn what is considered "good" or "bad" and what is rewarded or punished. Through natural and arranged consequences the environment teaches them to inhibit unrewarded or sanctioned responses and emit approved or rewarded ones. They also learn strategies for achieving what they have learned is desirable and rewarding (Harris, 1982; O'Leary & Dubey, 1979).

Behavioral theorists assign the major controlling role in behavior to the environment and propose that individuals learn to control their own behaviors to adapt to environmental constraints. From this perspective, both the goals for self-regulated effort and the means to exercise control come largely from outside the child. If the child behaves well or badly from the larger society's point of view, it is the learning or training environment that is at fault.

The Social Learning Theory Perspective

Social learning theory grew out of the behavioral learning theory of Clark Hull, in an attempt to account for the power of imitation in learning (Miller & Dollard, 1941). Bandura's (1977, 1986, 1997) social cognitive learning theory is preeminent today. It focuses on the cognitive aspects of social learning and gives weight to both internal and external (environmental) forces in controlling behavior. Both positive and negative social behaviors are considered the product of learning but internal interpretive and evaluative capacities allow a high degree of individual control.

Prosocial and antisocial behaviors and attitudes are learned from individual experiences of reward or punishment and from observing behavior and its consequences in others. There is some evidence that genetic differences such as gender affect the tendency to engage in both altruistic and aggressive behaviors (Bandura, Ross, & Ross, 1963; Rushton, Fulker, Neale, Nias, & Eysenck, 1986; Schunk, Schunk, Hallam, Mancini, & Wells, 1971), but Bandura's theory focuses on the importance of learning. He believes that behavior patterns are learned, remembered, and used because they have produced desired results.

With increasing age and experience, what is considered desirable is influenced by an individual's internal standards for behavior as well as the immediate external contingencies of reward and punishment in the environment. These internal cognitive regulators evaluate which behaviors are effective and appropriate in a particular situation. They also generate affect. An individual may reward herself (with feelings of self-efficacy) for living up to performance standards and punish herself (with feelings of self-contempt) for failure to do so, even in the absence of external contingencies or in opposition to them. The optimal outcome of social learning from this perspective is an individual who can distinguish socially approved right from socially sanctioned wrong behaviors and will attempt to act in accordance with these principles without the need for external rewards and punishments.

The Piagetian Perspective

According to Jean Piaget's (1965) theory, the "moral" development of the child depends on both cognitive development and interactions with others. He held that children's moral behavior reflects their level of understanding of the perspectives of others, the rules of society, and reciprocal fairness or "justice." His observations convinced him that young children do not understand the reasons behind social rules and the importance of intention in judging the morality of social behavior and the seriousness of infractions.

Piaget outlined stages in the development of moral thinking. During the first 4 years, children are in a "premoral" period with little understanding of what a social rule is or what purpose it serves. In playing games, for instance, they may make up rules unsystematically and change them arbitrarily when the game's progress or outcome does not suit them. At the age of 4 or 5, children enter the stage of "moral realism," in which their judgments of behavior are based on the amount of benefit or damage they produce. Intention is not considered, so a well-intentioned act such as helping another child carry a chair may be considered "bad" if it results in an accident with the chair such as bumping into another child's block construction and knocking it over. During this period children also see rules as absolute and unalterable. Differing circumstances and outcomes cannot affect the letter of the law, and there are no exceptions. At age of 9 or 10, Piaget proposed, children move into a stage of "moral subjectivism." They now understand social rules as somewhat arbitrary constraints that can be interpreted in relation to circumstances and altered by social consensus in light of more general moral principles of fairness and justice. Children are also capable of considering subjective motives and intentions in their judgments of behavior.

From Piaget's perspective, both moral judgments and the ability to control behavior in line with these judgments develop as the child becomes capable of logical thinking and understanding the perspectives of others. The development of social understanding is assisted by interactions with others, particularly peers who have perspectives different from the child's own. Differing feelings, wishes, and goals produce interpersonal conflict. This is translated into cognitive conflict as the child tries to assimilate the interpersonal events and deal with them effectively. Gradually, the challenges posed by social conflicts result in accommodations to the child's current conceptions and the development of more adequate conceptual models and strategies for action. As the child develops logical thinking, she begins to understand the principles of reciprocity and fairness.

In Piaget's theory it is assumed that the desire to engage in prosocial behavior accompanies the child's growing understanding of what is moral or right. There is no hint of Freud's aggressive will to destroy (*thanatos*) (Freud, 1955) or instinct-based self-interest (id) that inevitably conflicts with the interests of others (Freud, 1930). Both Piagetian and ethological theories emphasize the importance of adaptation; however, Piaget focused on the primacy of the human mind rather than instinctual tendencies coded in the genes to account for the adaptive process. It is the mind, rather than external patterns of reinforcement or punishment, that shapes the child's understanding of reality. The child's mind is also assumed to have an innate need to understand the world; evidence that conflicts with internal models of reality creates cognitive conflict. This conflict pushes the developmental process forward from inside as the child interacts with the social and physical environment. Both thinking and behavior are the products of these developing mental models of reality, so internally controlled moral behavior requires internally constructed moral principles of right and wrong, which change with age and cognitive development.

Table 4.1 presents a summary of the various theoretical perspectives on the source of prosocial behavior that have been described in the preceding sections.

RESEARCH ON THE DEVELOPMENT
OF PROSOCIAL BEHAVIOR

Overview of Research Evidence

The psychological research literature defines prosocial behaviors as voluntary behaviors that are intended to help or benefit others. Prosocial behaviors frequently examined in young children include sharing and helping (Rheingold, Hay, & West, 1976; Rheingold, 1982). *Altruism* refers to those prosocial behaviors that are induced by intrinsic motivation to help or be useful to others rather than by motivation for personal gain (such as being liked or accepted) (Eisenberg & Mussen, 1989). Altruistic behaviors studied in young children include comforting, defending (Zahn-Waxler, Radke-Yarrow, & King, 1979), and empathy (Eisenberg & Miller, 1987).

TABLE 4.1. Theoretical Perspectives on the Source of Prosocial Behavior

Theoretical perspectives	Source(s) of prosocial behavior
Ethological	Instinctual origins—"prosocial" behavior contributed to the survival of the species by inducing parental care, sharing resources with others, and reducing aggression
Psychoanalytic	Instinctual origins—(Freud) proposed that "life instincts" promote positive life-affirming, loving relationships with others and constructive work, and "death instincts" promote a tendency to destroy, including aggression Control mediated by: • *Freud*—superego, internalized at about age 5, has two parts: (1) conscience (internalized experiences of punishment), which controls behavior by guilt, and (2) ego ideal (internalized experiences that have been rewarded), which generates pride in living up to the ideal • *Neo-Freudian*—ego, with innate goals of competence, self-fulfillment, development of meaning and values, friendship, and unselfish love
Behavioral	Learned—positive social behaviors shaped by environmental contingencies of reward (reinforcement) and punishment Control mediated by environmental consequences of behavior and learned/remembered rules and constraints (providing promise of reward and threat of punishment)
Social learning	Learned—positive social behaviors and attitudes learned from individual experiences of reward and punishment, observing behavior and its consequences in others Control mediated by learned expectations of reward or punishment in the environment and internalized "performance standards" that generate self-reward when the child lives up to standards and self-punishment when she fails to live up to standards
Piagetian	Cognitive development—moral development depends on development of cognitive understanding of fairness and justice, which is related to the development of logical thinking Control mediated by the child's understanding of reciprocity and the perspectives of others

Research has suggested that the tendency to engage in prosocial behaviors is influenced by biological, cognitive, and cultural factors, with gender, personality variables (such as sociability), socialization experiences, and situational conditions making a difference (Eisenberg & Mussen, 1989; Hoffman, 1970a, 1982). There appears to be some consistency in prosocial behavior over different situations (Friedrich & Stein, 1973; Rutherford & Mussen, 1968; Strayer, Wareing, & Rushton, 1979) and some stability in prosocial tendencies over time in young children (Baumrind, 1971). Summarizing a large body of research on prosocial behavior in children, Eisenberg and Mussen (1989) conclude that children are most likely to help, share with, and comfort others when they are "relatively active, sociable, competent, assertive, advanced in role taking and moral judgment, and sympathetic." They suggest that the parents of these children are "likely to combine nurturant, supportive parenting practices with modeling of prosocial acts, discussions of the effects of such acts for others, inductive disciplining, expectations of mature behavior, and early assignment of responsibility for others" (p. 151).

Researchers have also attempted to document associations among a variety of positive and negative social behaviors and outcomes. Connections have been found between perspective taking and altruism (Iannotti, 1978; Underwood & Moore, 1982; Staub, 1971) and between prosocial behaviors and both social competence (Dodge et al., 1986; Katz & McClellan, 1997) and peer acceptance (Howes, 1988). Relationships between aggression and lack of perspective-taking skill (Chandler, 1973), lack of social competence (Eisenberg et al., 1993), and peer rejection (Achenbach & Edelbrook, 1981, 1991) have also been found.

Prosocial Behaviors in Infants and Toddlers

Social awareness can be observed in early infancy. From birth, infants pay particular attention to patterns and shapes that resemble faces and to sounds in the frequency of the female human voice. They also show a striking awareness of the social responses of others. As early as 2 months of age they distinguish a person who intends to communicate with them from a person who is talking to someone else, and are particularly aware of the actions and expressions of other people (Dunn, 1988). By the time they are 8 months old, infants are sensitive to the direction of gaze of another person and can follow it (Scaife & Bruner, 1975). They are also able to distinguish different emotional reactions in adults (Klinnert, Campos, Sorce, Emde, & Svejda, 1983). They appear to be interested in others' feelings as well as in what they are doing (Gelman & Spelke, 1981) and respond with "global empathy" to the distress of other infants, acting as though what happens to another is happening to themselves (Hoffman, 1987).

Toddlers demonstrate a more advanced understanding of others and of social rules. They respond more clearly to other people's distress and may attempt to comfort them (Zahn-Waxler & Radke-Yarrow, 1982; Zahn Waxler, Radke-Yarrow, Wagner, & Chapman, 1992). They also become increasingly aware of adult standards and show uncertainty or distress when these standards are violated (Emde, Biringen, Clymann, & Oppenheim, 1991; Stipek, Recchia, & McClintic, 1992). By the end of the second year toddlers use social referencing—particularly checking the mother's or primary caregiver's reactions—to evaluate behaviors and are responsive to negative affective signals from others (Emde, 1992). They show distress or "deviation anxiety" when they perform or are about to perform a forbidden behavior (Hoffman, 1985; Kochanska, 1993). In addition, 2-year-olds spontaneously correct forbidden actions, often accompanying this behavior with self-directive language such as "No, no" or "Can't" (Londerville & Main, 1981). They may verbally express concern or even attempt reparation for mistakes, such as trying to wipe up spilt juice (Cole, Barrett, & Zahn-Waxler, 1992).

Toddlers also begin to demonstrate "shame" when they are caught in transgressions of social rules (Erikson, 1963). Their sense of right and wrong is based on external standards, and their compliance with these standards usually requires the presence of an adult. They can begin to control sanctioned behaviors, but social rules are not yet internalized so they do not yet operate as inner prohibitions. Toddlers do, however, engage in a variety of spontaneous prosocial behaviors.

Spontaneous prosocial behaviors such as helping or sharing are demonstrated by children as young as 18 months (Rheingold et al., 1976; Rheingold, 1982). Without prompting or reward they may be willing to give or share toys with others. They may also spontaneously join an adult in household chores, sometimes specifying their intention by using the word "help" as they begin to work. Rheingold (1982) suggests that these are "natural" behaviors that grow out of young children's interest in people and their activities and their desire to imitate and join in.

Evidence of prosocial tendencies in young children are equally evident in their responses to other people's distress. They show evidence of true empathy early in the second year (Zahn-Waxler et al., 1979), and their emotional responsiveness and attempts to comfort or even defend others in distress increases with age (Zahn-Waxler & Radke-Yarrow, 1982). The research on empathy is complex, but a variety of studies suggest that the ability to empathize with distress in others is related to altruistic behavior (Eisenberg & Miller, 1987).

Hoffman (1987) outlines stages in the development of empathy from the first year to late childhood. He suggests that before infants can differentiate themselves from other people, they are incapable of true empathy. They cry when others cry from "contagion" or from involuntary global reactions. As the distinction between self and other becomes clearer, the child's feelings of empathy become more sophisticated and altruistic caring is increasingly involved. There is evidence that higher levels of early empathy and prosocial or altruistic behaviors predict similar positive behavior patterns at the age of 7 (Zahn-Waxler & Radke-Yarrow, 1982).

In a series of three longitudinal studies, Judy Dunn (1988) observed the behaviors of 1- to 3-year-old children in the natural environment of their homes. She argues that during this period children develop powers of social and moral understanding that they use to understand themselves, their goals, their emotional experiences, and their relationships with others, especially with those in their families. Her observations suggest that children are interested in and concerned about the distress of their mother and siblings early in the second year. By the latter half of that year they are capable of making sympathetic attempts to comfort these family members. In the third year their efforts to comfort "reveal a more sophisticated grasp of how the other's distress might be alleviated—with distraction, affection, humor, or the aid of adults" (p. 105). These efforts are spontaneous and self-directed and reveal a higher level of social understanding than is usually attributed to toddlers.

Dunn's work also reveals similar prosocial tendencies and understandings in relation to sharing. At 18 months of age toddlers were able to understand when a sibling wanted what they had and would sometimes offer to share before being asked. By the third year they "not only recognize what the other wants but have grasped the idea that sharing is often expected (especially if it is food) and use this as one justification for their own demands" (1988, p. 106). Dunn notes that in her sample of children, spontaneous (self-directed) sharing with siblings often involved self-sacrifice and was relatively rare. Providing comfort to parents or siblings required less or no sacrifice and was more frequent.

Dunn's (1988) longitudinal studies also investigated the development of cooperation between siblings. She found that in both the second and third years toddlers were "willing cooperators in play, picking up the mood of the sibling, coordinating their own actions to those of the sibling, taking roles complementary to those of the sibling, and by two years old sharing the collective symbolism of a pretend world. In the context of play, the children *helped* toward achieving a mutual goal" (p. 125). At the older end of this age range, children were very active in joint activities and were able to initiate innovative suggestions about what should be done in the play episodes.

Dunn stresses the interdependence of cognitive, emotional, and motivational factors in the development of social understanding. She also comments that although children at these young ages cannot talk about moral judgments in situations in which they are not involved, their actual behavior reveals a surprising amount of social and moral understanding. From the age of 18 months,

> [They] understand how to hurt, comfort, or exacerbate another's pain; they understand the consequences of their hurtful actions for others and something of what is allowed or disapproved behavior in their family world; they anticipate the response of adults to their own and to others' misdeeds; they differentiate between transgressions of various kinds. They comment and ask about the causes of others' actions and feelings. (p. 169)

Dunn proposes that, to some extent, toddlers understand others' feelings, understand others' goals, understand social rules, and (in the course of the third year) understand others' minds (pp. 169–173).

Noting the relationship between children's sense of self and their feelings of "efficacy" and "being a cause," Dunn argues that a positive self-concept in relation to management of social relationships "should not be equated with the satisfaction of self-interest at the expense of the interests of others" (p. 178). She contends that children have an innate or early sense of relatedness to others and that concern for others is not separable from concern for the self. From her perspective, it is not so much the guilt and fear experienced when they fail to live up to standards (as suggested by Hoffman, 1976, 1983) that leads children to control inappropriate or unacceptable behavior and engage in prosocial or altruistic actions. Rather, it is the child's enjoyment of positive experiences with others and a desire to behave in ways that increase the probability that these experiences will occur. This view is echoed in Emde and Buchsbaum's (1990) proposal—that it is not autonomy *or* connectedness that is the issue for toddlers, but autonomy *with* connectedness.

Importance of Experience

Social interest and responsiveness appears to be innate in young children, but the social environment influences the way this interest and responsiveness develops. Babies are highly social and need social interaction as well as physical caregiving from others (Sroufe, 1995). Responsive caregiving appears to increase the child's "investment" in human relationships and her desire to learn about and comply with the "ways and rules" of her social world (Ainsworth, Bell, & Stayton, 1974; Kochanska, 1993). Sroufe (1995) describes this process as "socialization from the inside" (p. 210).

The modeling provided by important people in the young child's environment also influences development. Prosocial and altruistic behaviors show little consistency over time and situations during the first 2 or 3 years (Hay, 1994), but research suggests that it is during this period of relative instability that the child is especially susceptible to environmental influences (Robinson, Zahn-Waxler, & Emde, 1994). Studies carried out by Zahn-Waxler, Radke-Yarrow, and their colleagues (Zahn-Waxler et al., 1979; Robinson, Zahn-Waxler, & Emde, 1994) have found that specific types of parental behaviors are associated with the development of prosocial behavior in young children:

1. *The provision of clear rules and principles.* Clear and explicit rules of behavior ("You don't bite people!") with clearly described consequences of actions ("If you hit Mary, it will hurt her") are more likely to foster prosocial behavior. These rules provide guidelines that the child can transfer to other situations. Simple prohibitions such as "Stop it" or "No" or "Don't do that" are not transferable.

2. *Emotional conviction on the part of the parent.* Rules and explanations should *not* be delivered in a calm and cool manner. The basic cognitive message should be intensified by expressions of strong feeling so that the child appreciates the importance of the message. Parents who presented rules in this way had children with higher rates of altruistic behaviors.

3. *Attributing prosocial qualities to the child.* When children are frequently told that they are "helpful" or "kind" or "generous," they internalize these attributions and try to live accordingly. They also begin to understand that motivation and control of actions in social situations comes from inside themselves and that they are responsible for what they do. When control is perceived to be external, children are less likely to be "good" when external monitors are removed.

4. *Modeling by the parent.* Modeling prosocial and altruistic behavior to children, especially by people who are very important to them, is a powerful way of teaching them. Actions may be even more effective than words with young children.

5. *Empathetic caregiving to the child.* A warm and responsive relationship between parents and children may be the most important promoter of prosocial behavior. It may account for the relationship researchers have found between secure attachments in infancy and later empathy with others (Waters, Wippman, & Sroufe, 1979). The social "climate" in which the child grows up has a major influence on the child's feelings about other people.

Although there is no magic formula that guarantees the production of prosocial dispositions and behavior in children, the five strategies listed here appear to increase the probability that their self-directed activities will include these tendencies. The emphasis on cooperation in these strategies echoes the findings of other studies that suggest children do not need to be forced to comply with alien standards. Rather, they need to be shown the standards and supported in their own attempts to comply with them (Kochanska, 1993; Maccoby, 1980; Waters, Kondo-Ikemura, & Richters, 1990). The strategies suggested by Zahn-Waxler, Radke-Yarrow, and their colleagues are relevant to the whole child-rearing period; however, the earliest years may be formative. Children's expectations about themselves and others may be increasingly hard to change as they grow older. In addition, their own behavior produces consequences and expectations in others around them that help to sustain early behavior patterns.

Prosocial Behaviors in Preschool and Primary School Children

The nature and organization of children's prosocial behavior changes during the preschool and primary school years with the acquisition of more sophisticated cognitive abilities. At ages 3, 4, and 5, children can talk about mental states such as thinking, remembering, and believing (Johnson & Wellman, 1982; Shatz, Wellman, & Silber, 1983) and are developing a growing understanding of "other minds" (Johnson & Wellman, 1982; Wellman, 1985; Wellman & Estes, 1986). They also try out a variety of roles and perspectives in sociodramatic play.

Children at 6, 7, and 8 years of age have more advanced role-taking skills that enable them to differentiate their own mental states from those of others more clearly (Piaget, 1965). They also have improved memory abilities (Case, 1985; Hoffman, 1983), internalized language for self-regulation (Berk, 1992; Vygotsky, 1962), and a greater capacity for reflection and self-monitoring (Case, 1985; Das, 1980, 1984). These skills allow them to adhere to social rules and responsibilities more reliably. In a number of non-Western societies, children in this age range are considered to have gotten "sense" enough to be given chores (such as child minding or cattle herding) to carry out independently (Whiting & Edwards, 1988; Whiting & Whiting, 1975). In Western societies, children are considered to "know right from wrong" or to have developed a conscience by the age of 6 or 7. They are held accountable for their actions in ways that preschool children are not and are expected to perform increasing numbers of activities independently.

Research has also suggested a reliable relationship between social cognitive and affective perspective taking and altruism (Underwood and Moore, 1982). This relationship underlines the importance of integrating both cognitive and affective factors when considering the development of prosocial behavior. In the past, psychologists focused on the cognitive limitations of preschool children and characterized them as relatively demanding and self-centered (Grusec & Lytton, 1988). More recent research (as described in the preceding section on toddlers) has shown that role-taking and empathetic abilities, which are assumed to be essential for prosocial and altruistic behavior, emerge much earlier in development. The more advanced role-taking skills of preschool and primary school children support more differentiated and conscious prosocial and altruistic activities (Hoffman, 1984).

With increasing age, the relationship between empathy and altruistic behavior becomes more predictable (Eisenberg & Miller, 1987) and individual differences in overall prosocial behavior become more stable (Eisenberg & Mussen, 1989; Hay, 1994). In 3- to 6-year-old children, research studies have found significant intercorrelations among giving, cooperating, sharing, helping, and comforting behaviors (Dunn & Munn, 1986). In 6- and 7-year-olds, instances of offering help, offering support, and making responsible suggestions to others were significantly intercorrelated (Whiting & Whiting, 1975). These behaviors were also highly correlated with teacher ratings of overall "altruism" and negatively correlated with "dominance seeking" (Krebs & Sturrup, 1982). In an extensive review of the relevant research, Eisenberg and Mussen (1989) conclude that "children's prosocial dispositions show appreciable degrees of consistency across situations and stability over time" (p. 22). There appears to be a relatively coherent and consistent disposition toward these behaviors in some children. This argues against a purely behavioral or "situational ethics" explanation for the occurrence of prosocial behaviors in children.

Preschool and elementary school children with strong prosocial dispositions are more likely to be well adjusted, good at coping, and self-controlled (Eisenberg & Mussen, 1989). This suggests that at least some negative or antisocial activity is the result of poor self-regulatory skills. As a child grows older, a disposition to act in prosocial (or antisocial) ways appears to become incorporated into the child's cognitive and affective view of the social world and of herself, where it can support conscious and self-directed motivation to engage in positive (or negative) social behaviors.

Importance of Experience

Eisenberg and Mussen (1989) suggest seven categories of determinants or antecedents of prosocial behavor: (1) biological, (2) group membership or culture, (3) socialization experiences, (4) cognitive processes, (5) emotional responsiveness, (6) personality and personal variables (such as sociability and gender), and (7) situational conditions and circumstances (p. 32). Although researchers have found evidence of genetically based differences in temperament and personality characteristics associated with prosocial behavior and altruism, such as sociability and empathy (see Eisenberg & Mussen, 1989, for a summary), environment appears to play the more important role. Environmental and genetic factors work together and in interaction to shape behavior, and there is abundant evidence that both social experiences and situational factors affect children's tendencies to behave in prosocial ways.

Oliner and Oliner (1988) summarize research on the family socialization techniques experienced by people who were altruistic as adults. Parents of these adults tended toward leniency with children but used reasoning techniques and set high standards of caring for others. They modeled and communicated caring values and rarely used physical punishment. They had close and caring family relationships, which helped their children internalize the family value for caring and for personal integrity. This description of family socialization practices is similar to those suggested by the research of Zahn-Waxler, Radke-Yarrow, and their colleagues (described earlier), which supports the development of prosocial and altruistic behavior in children.

Generalizing from a large body of research, Hoffman (1983) also suggests similar techniques for nurturing the development of an internal motive of caring for others in children. He supports the importance of giving reasons for social rules and the use of induction. For younger children, he suggests providing simple cause–effect reasoning ("If you push him, he will fall down and cry"), followed by statements clarifying a victim's feelings or intentions ("He was not trying to take your toy, he only wanted to play with you"). When children are older Hoffman proposes, more subtle psychological reasons and effects can be provided ("She is sad because she wants to be your friend and you wouldn't let her join the game"). Acts of reparation can also be suggested ("If you give back his toy, he will feel better") and moral lessons drawn ("Everyone should be given a turn"). Using an information-processing model, Hoffman contends that it is "(a) the mix of parental power, love, and information, (b) the child's processing of the information in discipline encounters and afterward, and (c) the cognitive and affective products of that processing that determine the extent to which the child acquires an internal motive to consider others" (p. 269).

Cross-cultural research from a study of six cultures (Whiting & Whiting, 1975) revealed that the rate of altruism observed in children was associated with the number of tasks assigned to children, the mother's work responsibilities outside the home, and the size of the family. In communities that assign many tasks to children (especially the care of younger children), that expect mothers to spend much time working in the fields, and where the size of the family makes it important for older siblings to help, altruism was highest. Socialization pressure in these societies is toward effort for the common good, and it is apparently clear to children that their help is needed for the welfare of the family.

Peer influences are also important in the development of prosocial behavior. Both positive and negative peer behaviors are imitated (Bandura, 1973, 1977) so peers can exert both positive and negative influences. Peers can sometimes be effective reinforcers of prosocial behaviors, such as sharing and helping, because they often respond positively to such behaviors (Eisenberg, Cameron, Tryon, & Dodez, 1981). Hoffman (1983) presents a more pessimistic evaluation of the effects of unsupervised peer interaction on the development of positive social behaviors. He suggests, however, that when peers from "homes in which inductions are frequently used" interact, the beneficial effects of constructive conflict described by Piaget (1965)—a decline in egocentrism and growth in the ability to take the perspective of another—may occur. He also suggests the value of indirect adult supervision, such as "stage setting" or "coaching," for peer interaction. This is similar to Vygotsky's concept of optimal support for learning administered by a person more skilled than the child (Berk & Winsler, 1995). Jerome Bruner and his colleagues called this kind of assistance "scaffolding" (Wood et al., 1976).

School and teacher effects on prosocial learning and behavior have also been investigated. Preschool teachers can strengthen children's prosocial response tendencies by modeling prosocial behaviors, by calling attention to children's own prosocial statements, by giving explicit instructions about sharing, helping, and the like, and by rewarding these behaviors when they occur (Eisenberg & Mussen,

1989). Their role is similar to that of parents in some respects, but their power to influence may be somewhat less because of children's strong attachment to parents.

Some types of teaching techniques and school programs have also been associated with increases in prosocial behaviors. A number of teachers use "cooperative learning" techniques in which children work together in learning tasks. The goal typically is to reduce negative aspects of competition and promote cooperation, interdependence, and helping, as well as increase learning and motivation. Research with older children (sixth grade) found that tension and conflict were significantly reduced and prosocial behaviors, such as cooperation and helping, were significantly increased in classrooms that used this approach. Performance in academic tasks, thinking skills, and motivation were also higher in these children than in a comparison group that had not experienced the cooperative learning approach (Hertz-Lazarowitz & Sharan, 1984). Younger children have less developed social and cognitive skills, so their participation in cooperative learning groups may have to be carefully monitored and scaffolded by adults.

A comprehensive longitudinal program to increase the prosocial behaviors and values of children from kindergarten to fourth grade was attempted over a 4-year period in several schools in a middle-class community near San Francisco (Solomon, Watson, Schaps, & Battistich, 1990). The program had five components:

1. Children engaged in cooperative activities similar to cooperative learning activities.

2. Developmental discipline techniques were used, which emphasized intrinsic motivation for academic excellence, prosocial values, self-control and commitment to rules and values, warm teacher–child relationships, discussion of moral principles, and student participation in decision making.

3. Efforts were made to promote social understanding by the use of discussions that explored different perspectives and feelings.

4. Modeled prosocial acts (kindness, responsibility, sharing) observed in teachers, other students, and characters in stories were highlighted and discussed.

5. Helping activities were encouraged in the school.

During the first 5 years of school, children in this program consistently engaged in more prosocial behavior than children in three equivalent comparison schools, and their social-problem–solving strategies included less aggression, more planning (reflecting internal control), more compromise, and more concern for the needs of others. There are interesting similarities between the San Francisco school program and the strategies for parents suggested by the Zahn-Waxler and Radke-Yarrow research (Zahn-Waxler et al., 1979; Robinson et al., 1994). They each have an emphasis on *both* cognitive understanding *and* emotional involvement and commitment. In addition, they both stress the importance of a warm and caring "climate," and the importance of modeling desired behaviors as well as talking about them.

Television viewing by young children has been associated with both positive and negative effects, depending on the content of the programs watched. Programs that model violence and antisocial behavior are associated with increased aggression in younger children (Friedrich-Cofer & Huston, 1986) and (in longitudinal studies) to an increased probability of aggression and involvement in crimes later in life (Eron, 1987). Friedrich and Stein (1973) also found that 3- to 5-year-old children who watched programs that model prosocial behaviors (such as *Mr. Rogers' Neighborhood*) were more likely to exhibit positive social behaviors and greater self-control than those who watched "neutral" or aggressive programs (such as those featuring Batman and Superman).

Table 4.2 summarizes the development of self-regulated prosocial behavior, and general effects of the environment on this development, in each of the four age ranges considered in this chapter.

SUMMARY

Parents, teachers, and the general public are interested in increasing prosocial behaviors and decreasing negative or antisocial behaviors in children. Determining what constitutes prosocial behavior across different social groups and settings is not easy because values and expectations about what is desirable or undesirable may vary. Understanding what promotes the development of a disposition toward positive social behavior is also difficult, because theorists have not

TABLE 4.2. The Development of Self-Regulated Prosocial Behavior and Effects of the Environment on This Development

Development of self-regulated prosocial behavior	Effects of the environment
	Infants
Innate interest in other people and in social interaction	Warm, responsive caregiving increases the child's investment in human relationships
Early awareness of and interest in feelings of others (global empathy)	
	Toddlers
Respond to distress of others and may attempt to comfort them	Adult behaviors that support self-regulated prosocial behavior include:
Engage in a variety of spontaneous prosocial behaviors (helping, sharing)	• empathetic caregiving
	• prosocial modeling
Can cooperate when activities are structured by an older child or adult	• provision of clear rules and principles with strong value for prosocial behavior expressed
Increasingly aware of adult standards and show uncertainty or distress when these are violated	• attributing prosocial qualities to the child
	Negative peer and media models may increase antisocial behaviors
Spontaneously correct some forbidden actions and show "shame" when caught in transgressions	
Usually need adult presence to exercise control over sanctioned behaviors (rules not yet internalized)	
	Prekindergarten and kindergarten
Are more able to control negative emotions and behaviors	Adult behaviors that support self-regulated prosocial behaviors include:
Can talk about mental states and has a growing understanding of "other minds"	• "stage setting" and "coaching" of appropriate peer interactions
Can try out roles and perspectives in dramatic play	• modeling and communicating caring actions and values
Have a greater capacity for independent cooperative interactions with others	• using prosocial reasoning to guide children's behaviors and emphasizing the effects of behavior on others
Are internalizing standards of behavior and more consistently act according to prosocial rules and values (if these are being internalized)	• avoiding physical punishment and criticism that demeans the child
	• attributing positive prosocial qualities to the child
	• giving the child age- and skill-appropriate responsibilities
	Negative peer and media models may increase antisocial behaviors

TABLE 4.2. (*continued*)

Development of self-regulated prosocial behavior	Effects of the environment
Primary school	
Have more advanced role-taking skills and greater understanding of the perspectives of others	Adult behaviors that support self-regulated prosocial behaviors include:
Have improved memory and ability to use language for self-regulation	• modeling and communicating caring actions and values
Have greater capacity for conscious reflection and self-monitoring	• promoting cooperative interaction, interdependence, and helping (more than competition) in learning activities
Are more reliable in adherence to social rules and responsibilities	• maximizing exposure to positive prosocial actions, principles, and values through exposure to live and symbolic (literature and media) models
Prosocial dispositions and values more conscious and consistent	• discussing positive and negative social experiences (live and symbolic) in relation to feelings, values, principles, and decision-making
	• giving age- and skill-appropriate responsibilities and expecting that they will be carried out
	Negative peer and media models may increase antisocial behaviors

agreed about how it develops. Some put more emphasis on innate tendencies, and some stress the importance of the environment in shaping both cognitive organization and behavioral responses.

Ethologists emphasize the continuity between animals and humans and point to the importance of certain types of prosocial or altruistic behaviors in the survival of the species. From this perspective, the bases for both positive and negative social behaviors are coded in the genes. Individual control developed because it aided survival, and behaviors that are now considered either positive or negative were "good" for the species at some point in evolution.

The psychoanalytic tradition accepts an instinctual base for behavior. Freud's interpretation of instinctual goals was somewhat pessimistic, often putting the fulfillment of individual needs in conflict with the needs of society. Recent formulations in this tradition have focused more on the social needs of the individual and the gratification of these needs through positive social contacts. In addition, there is a stress on distinctly human requirements for fulfillment and happiness such as competence, meaning, and values. Humans are also considered to be capable of unselfish concern for the welfare of others.

Behavioral theorists stress the continuity between humans and animals, citing the ability of the reward and punishment contingencies in the environment to shape their behavior. External rewards and punishments are assumed to account for the development of both behavior control and conscience. The child develops the ability to control impulsive behavior in order to reach desirable long-term or delayed rewards. There are no universal or necessarily "good" or "bad" behaviors. Conscience is the result of learned associations between the performance of forbidden behaviors and past punishments. Behaviors that have been rewarded in the past are associated with positive feelings and are more likely to be performed in the future. Children can also be trained to use specific techniques such as self-monitoring and self-instruction to enhance control of their own behavior.

Early social learning theorists added the ability to learn by imitation to the behavioral learning perspective. Bandura's more recent social learning theory focuses on the importance of cognition in observational learning. Standards for judging the effectiveness and morality of personal behaviors are internalized by children as a result of both individual experience and observing others. These "performance standards" also provide the basis for self-evaluation and individual control of behavior. Bandura has not suggested any universally applicable set of moral behaviors. His theory proposes a more relative and situational view of what is considered positive or negative behavior.

Piaget viewed prosocial or moral development as the product of both an increasing capacity for logical thinking and the accumulation of social experience. Logical thinking allows the child to begin to understand reciprocity and fairness and, ultimately, justice. Social experience provides exposure to the constraining rules of particular societies and, through interactions with peers that challenge her egocentric perspective, generate a growing appreciation of the perspectives of others. Piaget assumed that children will control their behavior in ways that follow their understanding.

Research studies have defined prosocial behaviors generally as those behaviors that help or benefit others, and altruistic behaviors as prosocial behaviors that are not motivated by personal gain. Investigations of prosocial behaviors in toddlers have suggested that these tendencies may have an innate base and that social understanding develops earlier than previously thought. The first 3 years of life also appear to be more important for promoting the development of prosocial behavior than previously thought.

A variety of associations among different types of prosocial and altruistic behaviors have been documented, and relatively stable individual differences in the tendency to engage in such behaviors have emerged in the preschool and primary school years. A number of studies have demonstrated that although biological differences have some influence on the development of the disposition to engage in these types of behaviors, the environment is more important. There is also some consensus on the types of environmental conditions that are associated with the development of prosocial behavior patterns. Warm and responsive relations with adults and a climate of caring, in which the value of caring for others is modeled, reinforced, and attributed to the child when relevant, seem to promote a prosocial disposition in children. Discipline techniques that provide clear rules and principles, describe the effects of behavior on others, and include adult expressions of feeling to highlight their commitment to the values expressed are also important.

5

Controlling Cognitive Processing

One of the most important areas children must learn to regulate is their cognitive functioning. They must develop the ability to exercise conscious control over their attention and memory processes. This control develops in interaction with the capacity to put the images of consciousness in sufficient order that they can support independent decision making and action. Children must organize information into categories and sequences that reflect and predict real-world experiences. They must develop rules and strategies for thinking and problem solving, and the ability to apply these to problems they encounter. They must also develop the ability to plan ahead, to monitor their progress toward goals and adjust their thinking and behavior accordingly, and, ultimately, to do this consciously and deliberately. Accumulating research evidence suggests that, to some extent, children spontaneously develop all of these capacities. Research also suggests that the environment can help or hinder their efforts.

Theories about the way children develop cognitive self-regulation have been proposed by both behavioral and developmental psychologists and by information processing theorists. Investigators have begun to use emerging models of brain functioning to address this issue, as described in Chapter 6. In addition, a large body of research has focused on children's cognitive performance and thinking processes. Both theory and research have documented age- and experience-related changes in children's ability to control attention and engage in self-directed thinking and problem solving. This chapter discusses a variety of different theoretical approaches and reviews the research evidence in relation to the four age groups of young children: infants, toddlers, preschool and kindergarten children, and primary school children.

THEORETICAL PERSPECTIVES ON THE DEVELOPMENT OF COGNITIVE CONTROL

The Behavioral Perspective

Although early behaviorists focused on observable behavior, increasing attention is now being given to the nonobservable behavior or "covert behavior" of thinking. Thinking is considered the behavior of the brain (Baldwin & Baldwin, 1998). Most of it is not conscious. Conscious awareness is focused on sensory impressions (from the five external senses and from internal sense receptors) and on an "internal dialogue" we humans carry on in our heads. This dialogue becomes possible when we learn language and then learn to talk to ourselves.

This view of the origins of thinking is similar to Vygotsky's (1962) theory about the relationship between language and thought. It is also closely related to B. F. Skinner's (1957) analyses of "verbal behavior" and Pavlov's (1927) suggestion that words provide a "second signal system" (available to humans more than animals) in associative conditioning. When language and self-directed thought are equated, verbal behavior in the form of external speech or internal thinking can be considered conditionable by the environment. Classical and operant conditioning principles can be used to shape the internal behavior of thought as well as observable behavior. Words are the "operants of the mind" and can be acquired and maintained by the same principles as external behavior operants.

From the behavioral perspective, children (and adults) learn to think from four sources (Baldwin & Baldwin, 1998):

1. They learn from *models* who transmit ideas through their actions and verbal communications ("It is really fun to go the circus," "I might catch a cold if I go out in this rain").

2. They learn from verbally transmitted *rules* ("Always start reading at the top of the page," "Good things come to those who wait").
3. They learn from *verbal prompts* that assist thinking at critical points when an individual cannot think of a word or phrase (" . . . April, June, and November," "His name is *Andrew*," " . . . 8, 9, 10").
4. Finally, children learn from *reinforcements and punishments* that can shape thoughts much as they shape other behaviors. They learn to think more frequently of things associated with rewards and less frequently of things associated with punishments.

Behavioral psychologists have described training techniques that assist children in controlling their thinking and problem-solving behaviors. Children can be taught specific strategies that apply to many situations, such as "Read (or listen to) the instructions," "Get all the materials you need before you begin," or "Pick up your toys when you are finished." Primary school children can be taught generalizable strategies for keeping track of their own responses (self-monitoring) and administering their own positive or negative consequences (self-reward or self-punishment) (Shapiro, 1984). Self-monitoring strategies include sets of (internalized) verbal reminders to the self, such as "Am I following directions?" " Did I do all the parts?" "Did I check all the answers?" Self-reward and self-punishment strategies also include internalized verbal evaluations of their own work, such as "I really worked hard on that," "I did a good job, because all my answers are right," or "My work looks messy." Children can even learn "self-shaping" techniques. They can be taught to evaluate and modify their own behaviors by comparing their step-by-step progress toward a goal with clear criteria for success at each step.

Children can also be taught strategies that apply to a narrower range of tasks. Examples include specific rules for spelling or grammar ("*I* before *e* except after *c*" etc.), sequenced steps for "carrying" in addition or "borrowing" in subtraction tasks, and specified procedures for science experiments. Behavioral theorists do not think that children invent or construct these rules, as Piaget suggested. The child must learn the rule and when to apply it from an external source. She must be trained to think.

Children can also be trained to pay attention to relevant information through the use of attention-focusing rules and strategies and reinforcement of appropriate attentive behaviors. They can learn to attend to teacher directions and to specific aspects of learning tasks and problem solving situations. They can be taught to use mnemonic devices to assist associative memory. Behavioral theorists do not assume that children search for the regularities of the environment and learn to take advantage of them. Rather, they assume that the environment shapes children's cognitive processes through direct teaching and reinforcement of appropriate responses.

Bandura's Social Learning/Social Cognitive Theory

Albert Bandura's recent writings (1986, 1997) focus on mechanisms underlying internal cognitive control of actions and thought. Although not denying the shaping power of the external environment, he proposes that in humans its influence is filtered and interpreted by a capacity for evaluation—of both the outside world and themselves. Individuals observe what is going on in the outside environment, their own actions within it, and the internal environment of their own minds. They are self-aware in ways that allow them to monitor and evaluate not only their ongoing behavior but also their own thinking processes.

Bandura (1986) identifies three subprocesses in the regulation of cognitive (or social or physical) activity:

1. Individuals observe themselves, in this case their own thinking and decision-making processes.
2. They judge the "efficacy" of these processes in reaching goals in the real world and against internal performance expectations.
3. They react to their own evaluations, attempting to modify or correct their cognitive activity when it is judged to be ineffective or inadequate in relation to their own internalized performance standards.

Evaluations of cognitive performance also generate emotional reactions that influence an individual's willingness to engage in similar cognitive activities in the future. Adults experience positive feelings of "self-efficacy" when their mental efforts are perceived to be successful in working toward or reaching goals *and* are congruent with internalized performance standards. They experience "self-contempt" when they fail in either arena. It is not enough to meet the standards of the outside world if they to not meet their own internalized standards.

Children have to develop internal standards for mental activity, the (metacognitive) capacity to monitor mental processes, and the ability to direct and correct them effectively. Bandura assumes that both maturation and learning are needed for the development of these abilities. Growth in children's capacity to understand language and make social comparisons and ability attributions, as well as increases in their knowledge base, contribute to the development of cognitive self-regulation (Schunk, 1989).

Children must also have both the maturity and the opportunity to learn, through modeling and instruction, to use each of Bandura's (1977) four cognitive processes in cognitive problem-solving situations.

1. They have to learn to *pay attention* to relevant environmental information and to their own cognitive processes.
2. They have to learn to represent and *remember* relevant information from the environment and from their own memory store. In addition, they must be able to remember a variety of relevant cognitive processing strategies and recall which of these strategies is likely to be effective in specific learning or problem-solving situations.
3. Children must also acquire the ability to *carry out* specific cognitive learning and problem-solving activities in particular cognitive tasks.
4. Finally, children must be *motivated* to carry out the cognitive activity, believing that they can be successful in doing so.

Very young children are not able to observe and evaluate their own cognitive processes. Training for (later) cognitive self-regulation in the early years focuses on modeling, verbal descriptions (of goals and how to reach them), social guidance (during tasks), and feedback (evaluations of the child's performance). Although the highest levels of cognitive self-regulation are not expected until adolescence, children can be taught specific strategies to help them regulate their own learning and problem solving starting in the fourth or fifth year and continuing more systematically when they enter elementary school (Schunk & Zimmerman, 1994).

As in Vygotskian and recent behavioral learning theory approaches, training focuses on verbal mediators. Children are taught "self-verbalization" techniques that function as self-instruction strategies to guide their cognitive problem solving. Modeled statements may include problem definition ("What is my goal?" "What is it I have to do?"), planning and response guidance ("What materials do I need to do this?" "What should I do first?" "I need to work carefully"), self-reinforcement ("I know how to do this," "I am doing this right"), self-evaluation ("Am I doing this in the right order?" "Have I made all the colors match?") and coping ("I have to try again when I don't get it right" "I need some help if I forget how to do it") (Meichenbaum, 1977, 1984; Meichenbaum & Asarnow, 1979).

There are some similarities in the training approaches advocated by behavioral theorists and social learning theorists who build on Bandura's theory. Both focus on the use of linguistically mediated strategies and the importance of reinforcement. However, Bandura puts more emphasis on the human capacity for self-observation and self-evaluation. *Internal* standards form the basis for a *self*-reward process that is at least as powerful as external rewards and supports self-regulation in cognitive as well as other areas of functioning. A person's perception and evaluation of her own performance guides her in self-regulation in the absence of (and sometimes in spite of) external rewards and punishments.

Vygotsky's Perspective on Cognitive Self-Regulation

Vygotsky's (1962, 1978) theory emphasizes the role of language and culture in the development of higher level mental processes and self-regulation. Both Piaget and Vygotsky held that children are active in their own development and develop in interaction with the environment, but Vygotsky saw the social environment as critical. While Piaget focused on the child's ability to construct the tools for logical thinking independently, Vygotsky proposed that the child was guided in these efforts by more experienced members of society.

In contrast to Piaget, Vygotsky believed that all higher mental functions, including voluntary attention, conscious memory, and logical and abstract thinking, originate in the social environment. He proposed that only "elementary mental processes," such as reactive attention and associative memory, are innate and appear without social assistance. These lower processes are also found in animals. In Vygotsky's view it is the "psychological tools" provided by culture that enable children (or adults) to master and control both the environment and themselves. These tools include language, counting systems, writing, works of art (and, more recently, computers), as well as specific strategies for attending, memorizing, and learning.

Acquisition of the psychological tools of a culture transforms the mind. When a child acquires language, she begins to think and remember in words rather than simply in actions or sensory images. Individuals who have acquired the tools of writing and reading or use television sets and computers think differently, according to this perspective, which emphasizes the context and means (tools) for thought. These tools are the products of culture and must be "co-constructed" with others and "internalized" by the child in interaction with others. As cultural and linguistic supports for thought are internalized, the child becomes capable of consciously and deliberately regulating attention, memory, and thinking (Vygotsky, 1978).

In Vygotsky's view the preeminent psychological tool or "mediator" needed to gain mastery over both behavior and cognition is language. He considered language the primary means through which culture is transmitted and the primary vehicle for thought and self-regulation. He believed that language is used for self-expression and communication with others before it is used for regulating thought and action. The speech of others assists the child in developing a cognitive understanding of the world and in learning to control her own cognitive activities. With accumulating experience with others, the child learns to use words as "external signs" in conjunction with external operations to help in the solution of problems (as in counting on fingers). The child also begins to use "private speech" (talking to the self) as a help in problem solving. Vygotsky observed that this kind of speech appears first at the end of an activity. With further development it shifts to the middle and then to the beginning of a task, where it takes on a (self-regulatory) directing and planning function. Vygotsky suggested that as the child reaches the age of 6 or 7 (the age when Piaget noticed that this kind of "egocentric" speech seemed to cease), egocentric speech becomes abbreviated and almost inaudible, then disappears as language "goes underground" and becomes internalized as "inner speech." During this period language becomes the primary mechanism for thought and self-regulation (Vygotsky, 1978).

Vygotsky thought that private speech helps develop thought by organizing behavior. As children label situations and their own activities within them, they are able to see recurrent patterns that might be hidden without the abstraction of language. Many situations with differing perceptual attributes can be labeled "dangerous" or "fun" or "school," and a variety of different situations can present opportunities for "sharing" or "climbing" or "building."

There is a growing body of research supporting the usefulness of language for assisting self-regulation in young children (Berk, 1992; Berk & Winsler, 1995). There is also evidence that learning can lead, as well as follow, cognitive development when adults or more competent peers provide guidance in the form of structuring or "scaffolding." They can break a task down into simpler components and provide hints, feedback, or demonstrations that enable a child to perform a task that is just ahead of her ability (in what Vygotsky identified as the child's "zone of proximal development"), then phase out these supports as the child develops the ability to perform the task independently (Wood et al., 1976; Rogoff, 1990).

In Vygotsky's view individuals cannot develop cognitive self-regulation without assistance from others. This assistance does not take the form of training or shaping, as in the behavioral approach. It involves the transmission of the psychological tools for thinking available in the culture through social interaction. The child is not passive in this transmission, but actively constructs her own version of what is being transmitted. The child's version is gradually modified in the direction of the mentor's approach in a process of "co-construction" of the tools for thinking and problem solving.

Piaget's Perspective on Cognitive Self-Regulation

The Swiss psychologist Jean Piaget studied biology and philosophy before becoming interested in psychology. He wanted to explain how the child's mind develops the ability to think logically and understand reality and saw psychology as a way the address this problem (philosophy's "epistemological" problem). Starting with the importance of self-regulation for biological adaptation, he proposed that the mind has cognitive correlates to the homeostatic processes the body uses to adapt to changing internal and external conditions. He suggested that children are intrinsically motivated to understand (mentally adapt to) the environment and that there are innate self-regulatory processes that allow them to do this in ways that reduce cognitive conflict and promote cognitive equilibrium. He also suggested that there are mental structures or "schemas" that store cognitive representations of reality and change in the process of adaptation (Piaget, 1967, 1970).

According to Piaget's theory, the innate "equilibration" processes of assimilation and accommodation that allow cognitive adaptation to the environment are intrinsically self-regulating. The child takes in information that she is developmentally ready to assimilate (fit into current mental schemas) or can modify current schemas to accommodate. The range of information that the child can accommodate is conceptually similar to that described by Vygotsky as the zone of proximal development, but Piaget focused on the child's developmental readiness to progress (notice conflict and accommodate) while Vygotsky focused on the environmental supports needed for progression.

Piaget believed that the environmental supports needed for the development of logical thinking exist in all cultures and that this aspect of development is universal. He thought that the child's mind is prepared or designed to discover the universal rules of logical and mathematical thinking. A child discovers these principles through everyday interactions with the physical and social environment without explicit teaching. Piaget believed that teaching is useless in this area of knowledge because each individual has to construct the necessary relationships inherent in logical and mathematical thinking in order to understand them. From this perspective, a child cannot be taught the principles of conservation or seriation or class inclusion; she must discover them. She must also discover important aspects of the physical world (physical knowledge) in interaction with it, rather than by being taught. The child is considered to be a little scientist—exploring, experimenting, discovering, and mastering fundamental areas of knowledge. It is only "social knowledge" (social rules and conventions) that must be taught, because they are arbitrary rather than logical and necessary or inherent properties of the physical world.

According to Piaget's theory, cognitive development is self-regulated from infancy onward because the equilibration processes are automatically self-regulating. The child is assumed to be active in constructing increasingly accurate representations of reality in order to avoid cognitive disequilibrium. The equilibration processes are similar to homeostatic mechanisms in that they automatically adjust to incorporate new information and maintain cognitive equilibrium. As the child develops the ability to cope with new information more effectively and her cognitive structures contain more adequate representations of reality, cognitive activity is more consciously and efficiently self-regulated and is less susceptible to mental conflict or disequilibrium. The development of the capacity for "preoperational" symbolic thinking during the preschool years, "concrete" logical operations at the age of 7 or 8, and "formal" operations (capacity for systematic and hypothetical thinking) at approximately age 12 provide significant stage-linked increases in cognitive flexibility and control over thinking and problem solving.

Neo-Piagetian Perspectives on Cognitive Self-Regulation

"Neo-Piagetian" developmental psychologists such as Robbie Case (1985, 1992) and Kurt Fischer (1980; Fischer & Rose, 1994) accept Piaget's belief in the child's active construction of knowledge and in structural changes similar to stages in the child's thought processes. However, where Piaget focused on the general (universal) aspects of development, their theories focus on "domain-specific" cognitive development and incorporate concepts drawn from information processing theory, such as limitations in memory, the development of "automaticity," executive control structures, and task-specific concepts and skills. They view children as problem solvers who acquire specific control structures and strategies for reaching goals. With maturing capacities (such as improvements in memory) and experience with certain kinds of problems, children learn to activate specific procedures or strategies to reach goals and to evaluate the effectiveness of the procedures used. They develop problem-solving strategies (procedures) through exploration and experimentation with objects and through observation, imitation, and interaction with others.

When mental control procedures are successful, they are stored (coded) in memory in ways that make them available for *voluntary* use in problem-solving situations. As the child matures, control procedures can become both voluntary and *conscious* and the child can reflect on and select strategies.

The Information-Processing Perspective on Cognitive Self-Regulation

Information-processing theorists build models of cognitive processing that attempt to explain how information from inside and outside the individual flows through cognitive systems in the brain. The computer is sometimes used as an analogy for analyzing human thinking, either through computer modeling of cognitive processes or through incorporation of computer terminology such as "storage," "feedback," and "executive routines." These terms suggest that the brain has processing routines that serve the same function as programs in a computer. Some of the processing routines (such as those supporting sensory integration) appear to be innate, and some (such as visual scanning procedures) appear to be learned.

Information-processing research is usually concerned with attention, perception, and memory and how these processes are combined in problem solving. Information-processing theorists examine individual and age-related differences in the way information is perceived, attended to, and remembered ("stored"/"encoded"/"represented" and later retrieved) in trying to solve different kinds of problems. A computer can take in more information, process the information more exhaustively and precisely, and store and retrieve information more accurately than human thinkers. Researchers study how children and adults deal with their limited processing capacities. They measure the time various processing procedures take and the amount of information lost during processing, and determine the types of errors that are made in retrieval.

Terms used by information-processing theorists to describe self-directed mental processing and behavior include *executive functioning* (Lezak, 1982, 1983; Luria, 1980; Walsh, Pennington, & Grossier, 1991), *planning* (Ashman & Das, 1980; Bidell & Fischer, 1994; Das, 1980, 1984; Delisi, 1987; DeLoach & Brown, 1987; Friedman,

Scholnick, & Cocking, 1987; Gauvain & Rogoff, 1989; Kirby & Ashman, 1984; Klahr & Robinson, 1981; Kreitler & Kreitler, 1987; Naglieri & Das, 1987; Miller, Galanter, & Pribram, 1960; Scholnick & Friedman, 1987; Wellman, Fabricius, & Sophian, 1985), using *strategies* (Bjorklund, 1990; Kirby, 1984; Siegler, 1986, 1988b; Siegler & Jenkins, 1989), and *metacognition* (Borkowsky, 1992; Brown, 1978, 1982; Brown & DeLoach, 1978; Duell, 1986; Flavell, Green, & Flavell, 1995). Although the scope of each term is sometimes defined to exclude the others, the terms are often used to label similar sets of somewhat overlapping self-regulation capacities. These concepts are described briefly in the following paragraphs.

Executive Functioning

In the neuropsychological literature as well as in information-processing research, executive functions include goal setting, determining a course of action (planning), carrying out the planned activities, and monitoring progress toward the goal. Executive processes are higher-level mental processes that control cognition and behavior. These functions are included in some definitions of *metacognition* (Brown, 1978; Flavell, 1978), but the psychological literature contains both terms. The emphasis in studies of executive functioning is on evidence of cognitive control, or lack of control, of activities, whereas the emphasis in studies of metacognition is on conscious awareness. Researchers studying mental retardation or brain functioning tend to use the term executive.

The executive system can break down at any point in the sequence of events that make up intentional, self-regulated activities. Breakdowns in executive functions have been investigated in studies of individuals with brain damage or mental retardation and have been attributed to problems in the frontal lobes of the brain (Das, 1980; Hebb, 1945; Lezak, 1982; Luria, 1980). Research has also suggested that the development of executive functions in children is related to development in the frontal lobes (an increased number of connections between brain cells and myelination of the neurons) and the growth of connections between frontal lobe areas and other areas of the brain (Case, 1992; Fischer & Rose, 1994; Goldman-Rakic, 1987, 1993; Stuss, 1992).

Planning

Another term used to describe cognitive self-regulatory functions in information processing theory and research is *planning*. Planning has been defined in different ways, but is generally considered to involve some form of internal predetermination of a course of action. Definitions may or may not include a conscious awareness of the planning process, and they may or may not include the ability to execute the plan. In an early definition, Miller et al., (1960) described a plan as simply a guide for action, with the ability to start, use feedback to correct, and stop behaviors, similar to the functioning of a computer program. More recent definitions have included the ability to represent a problem, set a goal, create a strategy or strategies to reach the goal, and monitor the process of working toward the goal (Scholnick & Friedman, 1987). Differences in definition are important for describing planning in early childhood. Although young children may not have a conscious and verbal awareness of their own plans or the planning process (Gardner & Rogoff, 1990), they do engage in overt goal-directed behaviors and may show some degree of awareness of their goals and the strategies they plan to use or are using to reach them (Bauer, Schwade, Wewerka, & Delaney, 1999; Cocking & Copple, 1987; DeLisi, 1987; Deloach & Brown, 1987; Goodson, 1982; Prevost, Bronson, & Casey, 1995).

Strategies

Strategies are sometimes distinguished from plans. Siegler and Jenkins (1989) differentiate strategies from plans by suggesting that strategies need not be conscious. They propose that strategies are goal directed, but that the same strategy may be used to reach a variety of goals and the same goal may be reached using different strategies. Some researchers have focused on strategies connected with specific cognitive skills, such as language acquisition (Maratsos, 1983), mathematics (Siegler, 1987, 1988a), and block building (Goodson, 1982), and others have suggested that strategies are usually domain or even task specific (Bidell & Fischer, 1994; Fischer, 1980). There is evidence, however, that in young children some strategies may be generally useful across tasks (Bronson, 1985, 1994; Prevost et al., 1995).

Although the term *strategies* is typically used to describe cognitive problem-solving activities, it has also been used to describe social information processing and goal-directed social behaviors (Bronson, 1994; Cirino & Beck, 1991; Crick & Ladd, 1990; Dodge & Coie, 1987; Feldman & Dodge, 1987; Shure, 1981; Spivack, Platt, & Shure, 1976). Specific strategies for entering a peer group (Putallaz & Gottman, 1981) and organizing social activities (Bronson, 1985) have been suggested. Social characteristics such as empathy and perspective taking have also been associated with frontal lobe (executive) functioning (Williams & Mateer, 1992), and social disabilities have been identified as the most distinctive characteristics of frontal lobe pathology (Dennis, 1991).

Metacognition

The term *metacognition* is commonly used in cognitive psychology. It refers to the ability to both reflect on one's own cognitive activity and exert deliberate conscious control over that activity. Metacognitive skills include being aware of one's personal knowledge base (knowing what one knows), being aware of one's individual learning, problem-solving, and memory capacities (knowing what one can realistically do), and knowing how to apply this knowledge in specific situations. Effective metacognitive control in a specific task requires a knowledge of the skills and strategies the task requires and a knowledge of how and when to use them.

Metacognitive awareness and control develop with age and experience. Preschoolers know that thinking is different from sensory–motor activities such as seeing and talking (Flavell, 1993). They may have a few strategies for approaching tasks (Bronson, 1985) and learning things they want to remember (Kail, 1990) and may be able to monitor simple tasks, noting and correcting errors. More sophisticated metacognitive knowledge and skills emerge after children enter school and continue to improve throughout the school years, perhaps as a result of school learning experiences (Duell, 1986; Flavell, 1979, 1993; Siegler, 1986). As children grow older, they become increasingly realistic about their memory capacities and limitations (Cavanaugh & Perlmutter, 1982; Duell, 1986; Flavell, Friedrichs, & Hoyt, 19970; Flavell et al., 1995; Markman, 1979), develop an increasing ability to use effective learning and memory strategies

(Brown, Bransford, Ferrera, & Campione, 1983; Kail, 1990; Siegler, 1986, 1989), and engage in more effective monitoring of their thinking and problem-solving activities (Baker, 1989; Baker & Brown, 1984; Flavell et al., 1995). Although young children do not have the metacognitive awareness and the resources for cognitive control available to adults, they are capable of intentional action and choice and are increasingly capable of cognitive self-regulation in pursuit of their goals.

RESEARCH ON THE DEVELOPMENT OF COGNITIVE CONTROL

Both the maturation of the nervous system and experiences in the environment are important in the development of cognitive control. As children's bodies and brains develop an increased range of abilities, they are better able to gather information from the environment and to cognitively cope with it. Physical development allows the child to interact and experiment more widely and effectively in the environment. The growth and development of the brain, in interaction with experience, support expanding representational, memory, and control capacities.

As children grow older, they not only have more information, they also organize it better and use it more effectively to reach goals. They learn what features of the environment they should pay attention to and what features they can ignore (because they are redundant or unimportant in their cultures) in order to make the best use of limited processing capacities. They learn how to use their memories more deliberately and efficiently, both for storage (encoding for later use) and retrieval (accessing information when needed). Using the organization and integration they are creating in their existing knowledge base, and learned strategies that help in storage and retrieval, children gain increasing control of their cognitive processing resources. As their pool of processing strategies becomes larger and more effective, they can manipulate larger and more complex bodies of information and engage in more complex thinking and problem solving.

As the higher level processing and control systems of the brain mature and children's processing skills become more sophisticated and efficient, they are increasingly capable of (metacognitive) reflecting on their own thinking processes. As they begin to be aware of and understand their own cognitive abilities and skills, they are more able to control them. The development of conscious awareness of cognitive processing, at about the age of 6 or 7, marks an important advance in cognitive control. Children can now learn to direct and monitor their learning, thinking, and problem-solving activities more reliably and independently. They can become "responsible" for their own learning and thinking, as well as their behavior, in significantly expanded ways.

Table 5.1 summarizes the theoretical perspectives on the development of cognitive control described in the preceding section.

THE DEVELOPMENT OF COGNITIVE CONTROL AND THE EFFECTS OF EXPERIENCE

The Development of Cognitive Control in Infants

During the first year of life infants begin to organize their experiences. They notice regularity and form categories—of speech sounds, faces, emotional expressions, colors, objects, and animals—even before they have words for them (Quinn, Eimas, & Rosenkrantz, 1993). They seem to be born knowing how to divide the world into categories (Gelman, 1998). Infants are also able to make inferences about the behavior of objects in the physical world and to differentiate these from the intentional interpretations they make about people (Karmiloff-Smith, 1995). They make causal inferences about their perceptions and the effects of their own actions (Corrigan & Denton, 1996; Donaldson, 1987) and are able to detect contingencies in both social and nonsocial contexts (Tarabulsy, Tessier, & Kappas, 1996). They develop expectancies about the behavior of objects and people and are surprised when these are violated (Bower, 1977).

The infant's cognitive exchanges with the environment change considerably over the first year, from a relatively passive and reactive involvement to an increasingly active exploration and search for patterns. During the first 3 months young infants gaze intently at faces and objects, especially those that are within the optimal range of focus for this age, approximately 12 inches from the eyes. They look back and forth from one object to another as if comparing them, and examine their hands in the same way. They continue to gaze in the

TABLE 5.1. Theoretical Perspectives on the Development of Control of Cognitive Processing

Theoretical perspectives	Development of control of cognitive processing
Behavioral	Awareness and control of thinking is mediated by language and is equivalent to an internal dialogue (talking to oneself) Children learn to think from models (who transmit "ideas" through words), rules (verbal maxims), verbal prompts (from others), and reinforcements and punishments (which "shape" thought as well as behavior) Children can be taught to regulate thinking with verbal strategies, self-prompts, and rules
Social learning	Awareness and control of thinking occurs through self-observation of own thinking and decision-making processes, judging effectiveness of these processes in reaching goals (in relation to performance standards), and correcting inadequate processes Children learn to think by learning to pay attention to relevant information, represent and remember relevant information, carry out learning and problem-solving tasks (and are motivated to carry out tasks, believing they can be successful) Children can be taught to regulate thinking by using "self-instruction strategies" (including problem definition, coping, self-evaluation, and self-reinforcement strategies)
Vygotskian	Awareness and control of thinking is mediated by language, which transforms the mind and enables voluntary attention, conscious memory, and logical and abstract thinking Children learn to think by "co-constructing" cultural tools (especially language) in interaction with (and mentored by) more experienced others; internalized speech (primate speech) enables self-regulation of action and thought Children can be taught to think through transmission of language and other cultural "tools" by more experienced others
Piagetian	Awareness and control develop as a result of cognitive development; increasingly complex and adaptive mental structures that organize action and thought are constructed by the child in interaction with the environment: • self-regulation is built into the equilibration processes (assimilation and accommodation), which allow incorporation of new information into existing structures and/or modify existing structures to accommodate new information when existing structures are not adequate Children learn to think by constructing increasingly adequate cognitive structures that organize and represent reality more accurately and support more complex and adaptive thinking Children can be taught social knowledge (social rules and conventions); physical knowledge about the world can be discovered; logical knowledge must be constructed by the child: • learning (accommodation) is precipitated by cognitive conflict, which causes cognitive adaptation • the ability to learn (and to control thinking) is linked to the child's age and stage of development

TABLE 5.1 (*continued*)

Theoretical perspectives	Development of control of cognitive processing
Neo-Piagetian	Awareness and control develop in domain-specific ways with the acquisition of domain-specific strategies for thinking and problem solving Children learn to think by learning skills and strategies to do specific types of tasks and solve specific types of problems; they can learn these through exploration, experimentation, observation, imitation, and interaction with others Children can be taught specific skills for specific tasks, and strategies that are useful for learning and problem solving in specific domains
Information processing	Awareness and control are mediated by executive processes (associated with the frontal lobes of the brain), which support control of attention and memory, decision making, goal setting, planning, using strategies, monitoring performance, and metacognitive functions Children learn to think by developing these functions with the help of experience and maturation of the frontal lobes (with accompanying increases in control of memory and attention) Children can be taught or can discover decision rules and specific strategies (for encoding, retrieval, organizing information, task attack, monitoring, and judging effectiveness of performance)

direction of moving objects that disappear, but do not visually search for them. During this period infants begin to discriminate and recognize recurring aspects of the environment. They begin to discriminate objects by color, size, and shape and recognize some familiar objects. They can distinguish a parent's face from the faces of other people if other cues of voice, touch, or smell are also available.

Young infants also begin to anticipate familiar routines. They begin to be soothed by the approach or voice of the caregiver before physical comfort has been initiated. Even if upset or crying, they may grow quiet at the cues that signal the beginning of a feeding routine before they have actually tasted food. They may become alert and focused as they recognize the beginning of a familiar social or object play routine and may anticipate steps in the routine with smiles or simple actions. As infants begin to anticipate and act in accordance with familiar patterns and sequences, they are showing the beginnings of the cognitive organization that allows control.

During the period between 3 and 12 months children have an increasing ability to detect predictive relations (Canfield, Smith, Brezsnyak, & Snow, 1997), as well as an expanding practical understanding of causal relationships and their own ability to be a cause (Piaget, 1952; White, 1960). They experiment with cause-and-effect sequences and show pleasure when their expectations are confirmed or when they are able to produce effects by their own actions. During this period children also begin to explore more actively the physical properties of objects and the behavior of people. They experiment with objects in a variety of ways—dropping them, putting them in and out of containers, and opening and closing doors and lids. They pay particular attention to the responses of people, observing their actions and reactions, and how others respond to their own behaviors.

During the period between 3 and 12 months children are increasingly able to focus and direct attention and to understand, predict, and experiment with the properties of objects (DeLoach & Brown, 1987). They can explore and control objects more and more deliberately, and they become interested in mastery activities (Jennings, 1993). While engaged in simple tasks, they are increasingly able to choose goals such as filing a container, opening pop-up or lock boxes, or fitting puzzle or construction pieces together. They are also learning to monitor the process of reaching goals, correcting mistakes and trying new approaches when they know or can invent them (Bruner, 1972; Fenson, Kagan, Kearsley, & Zalazo, 1976; Piaget, 1952, 1954).

Importance of Experience

The environment provides "food" (in the form of both stimulation/ arousal and content) for the growth of the mind. Although a child spontaneously notices regularities and forms categories and expectations, the cognitive categories the child develops, the causal connections and contingencies she notices, and the expectancies she forms depend to a large extent on her experiences with people and objects in her environment. Early self-regulation is shaped by the child's internalization of routines and cycles of stimulation in the environment (Als, 1978; Hofer, 1988; Kopp, 1982). Experience also shapes the way the child begins to sort out the environment and form concepts. Some types of people, objects, and events become more salient and noticeable as they are gradually infused with meaning from past experiences.

Caregivers are particularly important for early cognitive organization and development. The availability of sensitive, responsive adults supports the infant's exploration of the environment and formulation of coherent expectancies about the behavior of people. Caregivers also structure social and caregiving routines for infants and provide objects and opportunities for exploration. Their awareness of the child's interests and capabilities is critical for creating a facilitating environment for a particular child's development.

Children's beginning expectations about the behavior of people and objects are dependent on the types of behavior, objects, and events they encounter. In sterile or impoverished environments there is less information to build on, and the beginning construction of patterns and expectations will be similarly impoverished. When environments have few predictable events and few interesting sights, sounds, and objects to explore, children's categories and expectations for sequence and routine will be less rich. In disorganized or chaotic environments recurrent patterns and sequences may not be clear enough for the infant to discern. When an environment has little recurrence or coherence that the infant can detect, the formation of categories and contingency awareness may be delayed. Consequently, the child will be less able to develop a sense that the world is orderly and predictable and may be less likely to attempt to influence or control it. Generally, children's developing understanding of the world, and their active experimentation and attempts to master it, are dependent on the occurrence of coherent, predictable events and the availability of interesting people and objects that are responsive to their actions.

Cognitive Control in Toddlers

Children between the ages of 1 and 3 years have a passionate interest in order, repetition, and routine (Ames & Ilg, 1976; Ames, Ilg, & Haber, 1982; Caplan & Caplan, 1977; Gesell & Ames, 1974). As they cognitively organize their world, they look for similarities and differences and notice small details or variations from what they have experienced before. They begin to match and sort objects and to play with pattern, sequence, and order of size. When toddlers are beginning to actively try to classify and predict aspects of their environment, they do not want these aspects to change. They want things to be put in the same places and done in the same way—over and over again. They want to find things just where they found them before and to put them back in the same places. They may demand that songs and rhymes be performed in exactly the same way, that books and stories be repeated word for word, and that social and physical rituals be carried out in exactly the same sequence with no parts left out.

Children's memory and ability to represent past events improves over these 2 years (Kail, 1990), allowing a more deliberate approach to choosing goals and the means to reach them. Increases in both cognitive awareness and sensory–motor skill support a growing interest in goal-oriented mastery as well as exploration of objects and the environment (Jennings, 1993). Toddlers begin to monitor their progress toward a goal more actively, noticing and trying hard to correct mistakes (Bruner, 1972; Kopp, 1982; Piaget, 1952, 1954; Scholnick & Friedman, 1987). Starting with a trial-and-error approach, they gradually acquire simple, self-regulated action strategies (for stacking, sorting, matching, or fitting together, for instance) that they can use in a variety of situations. At these ages children are controlling their choices and problem solving in action; they are not yet planning ahead (DeLisi, 1987).

Significant advances in language development assist children's developing organization and classification of their environment. Toddlers use words to label classes of objects that have perceptual or functional similarity (Brown, 1973; Nelson, 1979). Researchers have found links between the acquisition of words for appearance and disappearance and the development of "object permanence" (the understanding that objects do not cease to exist when they are out of sight), and between the acquisition of words and the development of "means–end" strategies to reach goals (Tomasello, 1996). Kopp (1982) noted that young children's memories are best in situations where meaningful semantic cues are used and called to their attention. Early language may facilitate children's cognitive organization and control before it mediates self-control in social and emotional situations.

Importance of Experience

As is the case with infants, maturation and experience work together in toddlers to form the connections in the brain that support cognitive development (Shore, 1997). In increasingly active interaction with the social and physical environment, and with the special assistance language provides, the toddler develops the conceptual categories, expectations, and cognitive routines that allow increasing cognitive self-regulation and internal control.

Cognitive self-regulation depends on the patterns, categories, routines, and rules that the child's brain has been able to form from the material presented in the environment. Because not all children detect regularities in the same way and at the same speed, the specifications for a rich and challenging environment may be different for different children. For instance, some may need fewer changes or more repetition than others. An optimal environment for one child may be over- or understimulating for another.

It is important that the child's world be structured in ways that allow her to detect its categories and rules and to have experiences of successfully influencing or controlling people, events, and objects within that world. For toddlers, as well as for infants, the environment must be coherent and consistent in ways the child can detect and assimilate and must provide opportunities for her to notice the effects of her actions within it. Her growing interest in cause–effect relationships in the world (Jennings, 1993; Piaget, 1954), and in being a cause herself (Hunt, 1965; White, 1959), requires scope for experimental manipulation.

The types of teaching strategies and support for problem solving offered by caregivers are also important (Fagot & Gauvain, 1997). Vygotsky's (1978) emphasis on the importance of teaching in a child's zone of proximal development has gained some research support. Joint problem solving in which the adult provides just enough help for the child to move forward on her own may also assist both development and self-regulation (Berk & Winsler, 1995; Rogoff, 1990; Rogoff & Gardner, 1984). When sensitively offered at the child's point of difficulty, the strategies supplied by the caregiver may be internalized by the child and may later be used independently. In order to support growth optimally, careful observation is necessary to find the growing edges of the child's competence.

Cognitive Control in Preschool and Kindergarten Children

Preschool and kindergarten children's self-controlled cognitive activities are becoming more organized and goal directed, and they are in-

creasingly persistent and skilled in carrying out tasks. In interacting
with objects, their primary focus is shifting from exploration to an
interest in mastering a challenge (Stipek, 1996). They are beginning
to use strategies to reach both social (Bronson, 1994; Rubin & Rose-
Krasnor, 1992) and mastery goals (Bidell & Fischer, 1994; Bronson,
1994; Kuhn & Phelps, 1982; Piaget, 1950; Seigler & Jenkins, 1989)
and can use simple plans of action in the process of reaching them
(Brown & Deloach, 1978; Gauvain & Rogoff, 1989; Hudson &
Fivush, 1991; Nelson, 1986; Prevost et al., 1995; Scholnick & Friedman, 1987; Wellman et al., 1985). Children in this age range are
learning how to learn and how to solve the problems presented in
their environments. They attempt increasingly complex tasks independently.

As learning becomes increasingly self-regulated, it becomes increasingly intentional and resourceful and involves the independent
use of a variety of strategies. Some strategies are specific to situations
and tasks (Fischer, 1980), and others are more general heuristics
(Bronson, 1994). Task attack strategies share a number of characteristics. They (1) are deliberate actions performed to attain particular
goals, (2) involve both agency and control rather than simple compliance, (3) are selectively and flexibly applied, and (4) are often socially assisted tactics for problem solving that become independent
approaches, especially when related to academic learning tasks (Paris
& Lindauer, 1982). There is an increasing focus in the literature on
the importance of goal-orientation, planning, and organizational
skills in the development of competence in young children (Baker-
Sennet, Matusov, & Rogoff, 1993; Brown & DeLoach, 1978; Casey,
Bronson, Tivnan, Riley, & Spenciner, 1991; Gauvain & Rogoff,
1989; Kirby, 1984; Klahr & Robinson, 1981; Kreitler & Kreitler,
1987; Sternberg, 1984; Wellman et al., 1985). All of these skills require effective self-regulation.

Importance of Experience

Experience can support or hinder preschool and kindergarten children's developing self-regulation in learning and mastery situations.
When children are given opportunities for choice and experiment
and are allowed to learn from the consequences of these choices, they
learn to direct their activities more effectively (Piaget, 1973, 1985).

Too much adult control, especially with a reliance on rewards, coercion, or punishment, produces compliance rather than internal regulation (Lepper, 1983).

Language experiences appear to be particularly important for the development of cognitive control. When rationales and verbalized strategies accompany directions, suggestions, and behavioral guidance, children may learn to reflect on the reasons for their actions and guide themselves with "self-language." Such approaches have been suggested by behavioral psychologists (Baldwin & Baldwin, 1998), as well as social cognitive (Bandura, 1997; Biemiller & Meichenbaum, 1998) and cognitive developmental psychologists (Berk, 1994; Berk & Winsler, 1995; Vygotsky, 1962). It also appears to be important that strategies be offered as solutions to specific problems the child is engaged in trying to solve, rather than "taught" in the abstract. In this context they enhance children's feelings of control and motivate them to "construct" an understanding of the concepts involved, rather than inducing a perception of external control and requirement to simply follow directions (Pressley et al., 1990; Pressley, Harris, & Marks, 1992).

Experience in attempting and successfully carrying out cognitive tasks also influence the preschool or kindergarten child's developing interest and skill in goal-oriented mastery. When the environment does not provide opportunities for engagement in such activities, or children's efforts are frustrated because the challenges are not appropriate to their level of skill, interest in cognitive effort and control may be reduced and skills may not develop as quickly. Opportunities to carry out multistep mastery activities without interference, or, when necessary, with assistance that supports the growth of control and independence, help children develop self-regulated problem-solving skills. Opportunities to engage in activities that build on the skills and strategies in children's repertoires, and that encourage the expansion or extension of these skills to new tasks, help them to generalize process skills that support control and to view themselves as competent.

Cognitive Control in Primary School Children

Research conducted over the last 10 years has suggested that a major source of the differences between the highest- and lowest-achieving children in school settings is the degree to which they become self-regulators of their own learning. High-achieving children use a number of strategic skills, including goal setting, planning, self-monitoring, and asking for help when needed (Meichenbaum, 1984; Pressley et al., 1990; Zimmerman & Schunk, 1989). They behave in ways that often characterize adult experts (Bereiter & Scardamalia, 1986), revealing a structured knowledge base, an organized strategic approach to problems and tasks, and persistent effort even after failure (Dweck, 1986).

Self-regulating procedures, such as goal setting, can be used to organize an individual's approach to a task and can contribute to how the task is accomplished. Self-regulatory mechanisms may be combined with other cognitive routines to form a program for accomplishing a specific task (Brown & Campione, 1981). Harris and Graham (1992) have suggested that self-regulation abilities are important in academic settings because they allow students to become more independent, to increase their level of task engagement (which facilitates learning and may decrease disruptive or off-task behaviors), and to monitor and regulate their own performance.

Primary school children are developing the ability to *consciously* set goals, select strategies, monitor progress toward goals, and revise task activities as they are being carried out. This conscious awareness occurs because they are beginning to develop the metacognitive ability to monitor and control their own thinking processes (Brown, 1978; Flavell, 1978, 1979, 1993). This increase in cognitive control is accompanied by more resistance to distraction than is demonstrated by younger children (Holtz & Lehman, 1995).

It has been suggested that part of the reason for primary school children's increasing ability to carry out self-regulated cognitive functions may be the increasing internalization of "self-speech" that is occurring during this period (Berk, 1992). Preschool and kindergarten children are beginning to use language for self-regulation but are not aware of their own self-speech. By the age of 6 or 7 children have become aware of this capacity in themselves and others, and their self-speech is becoming internalized rather than overt (Flavell, Green, Flavell, & Grossman, 1997). They are beginning to think silently in words. Vygotsky (1962) proposed that internalized speech is a powerful vehicle of memory and thought. Others have suggested that it contributes to many aspects of self-control (Barkley, 1997).

Importance of Experience

Experience is important in the development of self-regulated learning and problem solving, and even in metacognition. Theorists have suggested the importance of independent experimentation with objects (Piaget, 1952, 1970), observation and evaluation of oneself and others (Bandura, 1986, 1997), and mentoring by those with more experience (Vygotsky, 1962, 1978). Cultural and environmental demands also appear to make a difference. Western schooling systems provide practice in using rehearsal strategies for remembering (Rogoff, 1986) as well as reflection on and correction of mistakes. The process of learning to read and write and the cognitive advantages of literacy may also make a difference (Donaldson, 1978).

As children become more self-aware during the primary school years, their perception of their ability to successfully control their own learning and problem solving becomes especially important and affects their achievement in school (Skinner, Zimmer-Gembeck, & Connell, 1998). Children's belief in their own competence and their ability to control the outcome of tasks attempted affect both the quality and the persistence of their academic efforts (Dweck, 1991; Schunk, 1991). Tasks that challenge children but that they can accomplish alone or with minimal help help them feel capable and in control. Even objectively competent children who doubt their own abilities may be less interested in school and perform less well (Miserandino, 1996). Responsive, positive, and contingent (on the child's behavior) interactions with parents and teachers, as well as the child's own experiences of success, appear to support the development of perceived control in children (Skinner, 1986).

SUMMARY

Many psychological theories have described how and why children learn to control their cognitive processing. Behavioral theorists have focused on strategy training, accomplished by teaching children to give themselves specific verbal instructions in cognitive tasks. Words, or "verbal behavior," are considered the "operants of the mind," to be shaped by the environment just as other behaviors are shaped.

Social learning theorists, especially Albert Bandura and his colleagues, who have focused on social cognition, emphasize the evaluative capacities of the mind. They propose that cognitive processing strategies as well as other behaviors are learned by observing and evaluating the behavior of both the self and others. From observation and the results of their own experiences, children develop goals and performance standards and use these to guide (control) and evaluate their own activities.

The developmental psychologists Lev Vygotsky and Jean Piaget both emphasized the child's active role in the construction and control of cognitive processes. Vygotsky and his followers have concentrated on the power of culture, and especially language, to shape the human mind. They have proposed that the cultural tool kit allows the child to develop higher level thinking processes, and that as development proceeds, language becomes the primary vehicle for thought and the means for self-regulation. They have assumed that the child actively constructs higher level thinking processes in interaction with more experienced members of society and actively strives for control and independence.

Piaget focused more on the child's independent ability to construct an understanding of certain universal properties of the physical world and of logical thinking through the innate adaptive processes of assimilation and accommodation. These processes are intrinsically self-regulating and allow the child to create increasingly effective and accurate cognitive representations of the world in interaction with the environment. Piaget emphasized those aspects of "reality" that he considered universal to all cultures. Neo-Piagetian theorists, followers of Piaget, have focused more on domain-specific aspects of development and incorporated concepts from information-processing models into their theories.

Information-processing theorists have attempted to chart how information from inside and outside the brain flows through cognitive systems and how these cognitive processes lead to independent decision making and problem solving. Their research has usually been concerned with attention, perception, and memory, how these processes are combined in problem solving, and how cognitive processing changes with development. There has been a specific focus on cognitive control systems that support self-regulated functioning. These include executive processes, planning, strategies, and metacognition.

Research on the development of cognitive control in young children indicates that both biological maturation and experience play a role. As children's nervous systems mature, they are better able to interact with the social and physical environment and to make use of information from these interactions. They not only gain more information but are able to organize and use it more effectively to solve problems in the real world. The attempt to organize and cognitively master the environment begins in infancy as children notice regularities and begin to form categories. During the first year they move from a relatively passive to an increasingly active search for patterns and contingencies they can manipulate. Responsive and predictable environments facilitate these developments.

Between the ages of 1 and 3 toddlers actively attempt to understand, predict, and control their social and physical environments. During this period of growing autonomy and developing language, children experiment with and test the limits of their world. They show intense interest in order and pattern and resist deviations from the expectancies they are beginning to form. The objects and events in a child's environment and the behavior of caregivers are particularly important for the development of cognitive control during these years. A balance between pattern and consistency (to facilitate an understanding of rules and routines) and responsive flexibility (that allows the toddler to influence and create effects on objects and people) appears to facilitate development.

Preschool and kindergarten children are gaining increasing cognitive control. Over this period, their focus shifts from exploration to mastery. They are better organized and more goal directed than younger children and have more strategies for carrying out cognitive tasks independently. The environment should provide appropriate opportunities for multistep activities and for choice, to allow practice in developing control. Children also appear to benefit from linguistically mediated strategies, offered when they need assistance in tasks they are interested in accomplishing. Assistance is most useful when it supports rather than supplants the child's own developing control.

Primary school children are developing a conscious awareness of their own cognitive behavior and can begin to make use of (simple) metacognitive control strategies. As they become more aware of themselves and their cognitive abilities, they are more vulnerable to perceived deficiencies in their cognitive performance and perceived lack of control, and this influences their academic performance. Positive and responsive feedback from others and the provision of tasks appropriate to their level of skill (so they can experience both challenge and success) appear to support primary school children's belief in their own cognitive competence and control.

Table 5.2 summarizes the development of self-regulated cognitive processing over the four age ranges and the major effects of the environment at each age.

TABLE 5.2. The Development of Self-Regulated Cognitive Processing and Effects of the Environment on this Development

Development of self-regulated cognitive processing	Effects of the environment
	Infants
Begin to organize experience: • notice and begin to anticipate regularities and routines • begin to form categories • detect contingencies and notice effects of own actions on people and objects • make causal inferences and experiment with cause-and-effect sequences Move from passive, receptive mode to active search for coherence	Appropriate levels of stimulation and coherence (regularity and routine, order and predictability) support cognitive organization Understimulating, overstimulating, or chaotic (unpredictable) environments impede the development of cognitive organization Responsive social and physical environments contribute to developing understanding of the controllability of the environment
	Toddlers
Memory improves Attention is more focused Language develops Choose goals and the means to reach them more deliberately Begin to monitor progress toward goal Move from trial and error to simple action strategies Actively look for order and predictability (notice small details and variations from previous experience, demand repetition and routine) Play with pattern, order (sorting, matching), and sequence (order of size, cause-and-effect sequences)	Cognitive organization depends on the coherence and predictability of the environment (patterns, categories, routines, rules, contingencies) A rich language environment supports cognitive organization Opportunities to engage in appropriately challenging (for age and skill) activities support the development of decision making, goal orientation, strategic approaches to experimentation and mastery, and early problem-solving and learning skills Teaching strategies that (1) provide assistance in the form of suggestions or strategies that can be used independently, (2) occur in the context of problem solving, and (3) intervene at the point of difficulty for the child are more likely to support self-regulated learning

TABLE 5.2 (*continued*)

Development of self-regulated cognitive processing	Effects of the environment
Prekindergarten and kindergarten	
Are increasingly interested in goals and mastering challenges Are increasingly persistent and skilled in selecting and carrying out learning and problem-solving tasks • are more organized and planful • use strategies to carry out tasks and solve problems • monitor progress of tasks more effectively and consistently	A rich language environment supports cognitive organization and self-regulation Opportunities to engage in appropriately challenging activities support increases in skills and strategies Opportunities for choice and experiment and being allowed to learn from the consequences of choice support the development of self-regulated learning and problem solving Too much adult control and/or reliance on external rewards and punishments reduces opportunities to engage in (and perhaps interest in) self-regulated activities Teaching strategies that (1) provide assistance in the form of suggestions or strategies that can be used independently, (2) occur in the context of problem solving, and (3) intervene at the point of difficulty for the child are more likely to support self-regulated learning
Primary school	
Show a marked increase in self-awareness Metacognitive awareness begins Speech is internalized and used for self-regulation (private speech) Have a more structured knowledge base and organized strategic approach to tasks Capable of conscious control of attention, some forms of planning, and use of strategies Have internal performance standards that guide self-monitoring and self-evaluation	Opportunities to have some control over choice of tasks and evaluate own progress support the development of self-regulated learning Opportunities to observe and be mentored by "experts" or those with more experience extend skills Appropriate levels of challenge (tasks that the child can control and master with effort or minimal help) increase the child's awareness of control and competence (and interest in self-regulated effort) Teaching strategies that maximize internal control and minimize perception of external control are more likely to support the development of self-regulated learning

6

Self-Regulation and Control Systems in the Brain

Research on the development of the human brain has increased dramatically in recent years as brain-imaging techniques have allowed noninvasive examination of both brain structures and active functioning. This research has focused particular attention on the early years of life as a time when the brain is developing fast and establishing many of the connections that support later development (Shore, 1997).

The human brain increases in weight from 300 grams at birth to approximately 1,300 grams at maturity. The brain increases in both weight and size for several reasons. First, the number of nerve cells (neurons) increases early in life. Second, more glial cells (which cushion and feed neurons) and capillaries are formed. Third, neurons develop more branches (axons and dendrites) and develop more connections (synapses) with each other. Fourth, a substance called myelin is gradually formed around neurons, coating and insulating them and increasing their speed of transmission. The lower parts of the brain (near the neck), which control breathing, heartbeat, and other life-support systems, matures first. The areas that support the integration of sensory and motor functions develop more gradually, and those that support higher level planning and metacognitive functions are not completely mature until adolescence. The frontal lobes of the brain are the last to be myelinated.

During development, connections form and strengthen between neurons and groups of neural "networks" that support specific functions. The brain forms more neurons and connections between neurons than will ultimately be used. Most of the extra neurons fail to develop connections and disappear before birth, but the remaining neurons continue to expand and to form branches and synaptic connections at a high rate. During the first 3 years of life the number and length of dendrites (nerve cell branches) and the number of synapses at points of connection between neurons increase to twice the adult level (Huttonlocher, 1993). The function of the cerebral cortex is considered to be closely related to the way these connections are formed. Stunted growth in cortical dendrites or defective development in regions of dendrites where synaptic contacts are located has been found in brains of mentally retarded individuals (Huttonlocher, 1993).

The "density" of connections in the young child's brain may account for both resilience and flexibility in early development. This massive "overwiring" appears to permit greater recovery of function after injury and greater possibilities for learning (Shore, 1997). The brain gradually loses connections it does not use, but the child's brain remains denser than an adult's brain until late adolescence. The period of greatest density is the early childhood years.

In addition to the development of connections between neurons and networks of neurons, there is also a "pruning" of unused connections. Brain communication routes appear to compete. If one set of connections is activated repeatedly, support and nourishment-providing mechanisms grow up around it. Connections that are infrequently or never activated lose their support systems and disappear (Edelman, 1992; Gazzaniga, 1992; Goldman-Rakic, 1987). With age and experience, brain connections become more numerous and more direct in areas that are stimulated. Connections that are not used are lost. The brain learns to perform activities required by the environment more efficiently, but it gradually loses plasticity and flexibility. As more connections are "committed" and others are lost, it becomes more "hard-wired." The early childhood period is the period of maximum flexibility.

The frontal lobes of the brain, especially in the prefrontal areas right behind the forehead, appear to be particularly involved in self-regulation (Barkley, 1997; Passingham, 1993; Rabbitt, 1997). Neurons in these areas form connections with many other areas of the brain and appear to be involved in the control of attention, working memory (Goldman-Rakic, 1992), and the regulation of emotions and drives. The frontal lobe areas are considered to contain the most advanced human functions, including those involved in planning, organization, and higher level executive control systems.

Research has suggested that the development of executive functions in children is related to development in the frontal lobes. This development includes an increased number of connections between brain cells in these areas, myelination of the neurons, and the growth of connections between frontal lobe areas and other areas of the brain (Case, 1992; Fischer & Rose, 1994; Goldman-Rakic, 1987, 1993; Stuss, 1992). Neuronal density in the frontal lobes increases more slowly than in other areas of the brain, and subsequently decreases more slowly (Huttonlocher, 1993). This density reaches a maximum between 12 and 24 months in the frontal area of the cortex (in contrast to a peak density at 5 months in the visual areas). It does not decline significantly until after age 7 and does not reach adult levels (50% of maximum density at age 2) until about 16 years of age. While density decreases with age, the length of dendrites in the frontal areas continues to grow—even into old age. "In general, a decrease in density of cortical neurons has been observed as one progresses from simpler to more complex cortical systems, both within a species and phylogenetically" (Huttonlocher, 1993, p. 119).

Synthesizing several models of frontal lobe functioning, Barkley (1997) proposes five "executive" frontal lobe functions that support self-regulation. The first executive function includes three *inhibitory* abilities: (1) the inhibition of automatic responses (that produce immediate consequences) in favor of responses that are more adaptive in the long run, (2) the power to interrupt ongoing activities when they are proving ineffective, and (3) the power to control "potential sources of interference that could disrupt, pervert, or destroy" ongoing executive functions (p. 102). This three-faceted executive system appears early and is necessary to support the other four functions. Eventually, executive inhibitory abilities include the power to control attention and inhibit distractions.

The remaining executive functions that support self-regulation in

Barkley's synthesis of other models are working memory, internalized speech, motivational appraisal, and "reconstitution" or behavioral synthesis. The *working memory* system allows the individual to recall past events and actively manipulate this information in order to anticipate and prepare for the future. Barkley suggests that this system allows the individual to plan, to engage in sequenced self-directed behaviors, and to modify future behaviors based on past experiences. He includes *internalized speech* in his model because research (Berk, 1992, 1994; Kopp, 1982) has documented its importance in self-regulated functioning. The *motivational appraisal system* provides for the "constraints . . . placed on decision making" by emotions and motivation (p. 104). The fifth executive system or function is the ability to *reconstitute* or synthesize behaviors—to "generate novel, complex, hierarchically organized, and goal-directed behavior." It includes the ability to "analyze or dismember past behavioral structures . . . then reorganize them into novel structures, sequences and hierarchies" in order to reach new goals or reach old ones more effectively (pp. 104–105). The five executive functions are interdependent and operate together to support self-regulation.

Frontal lobe areas are involved in both cognitive and social awareness and control (Dennis, 1991). They support not only cognitive problem-solving activities and motivation and goal directedness, but also complex social cognitions and behaviors—including a sense of self, the ability to understand others, and the ability to communicate with them (Dennis, 1991). Studies of children and adults with brain damage or deficits in frontal lobe areas have confirmed the critical importance of these areas in both cognitive and social self-regulation (Barkley, 1997; Lezak, 1983; Luria, 1980).

Damage to the frontal lobe can cause profound impairment in everyday life, even when many cognitive functions appear to be intact when they are tested in isolation (Denckla & Reader, 1993; Manly & Robertson, 1997). Executive functions in this area orchestrate an individual's activities to produce coherent and effective behavior (Luria, 1980; Shallice & Burgess, 1991). The frontal lobe is involved in maintaining attention (Manly & Robertson, 1997) and in working memory (Goldman-Rakic, 1987), which supports organizing and monitoring information-processing activities (Luria, 1972; Shallice, 1988). Children with executive dysfunctions exhibit disorganization, inattentiveness, and impulsivity (Denckla & Reader, 1993). They are also more likely to be diagnosed as having attention-deficit/hyperactivity disorder (ADHD) (Barkley, 1997).

This chapter examines research on the developing brain as it relates to the development of self-regulation in the areas of motivation, control of emotions and behavior, and control of cognitive processing. It also considers the importance of the environment in brain development.

BRAIN DEVELOPMENT AND MOTIVATION FOR SELF-REGULATION

As described in Chapter 2, many psychologists have proposed that human beings have innate motivation to understand, predict, and control their environments. From the first months of life infants appear to be rewarded by contact with people and objects in the environment, by recognizing and predicting events, and by controlling their own activities and the people and objects around them. They are surprised, especially attentive, and sometimes upset when their expectations are violated. Moreover, after experiencing successful control, they become distressed when their efforts to achieve it are unsuccessful. Under favorable conditions the child moves from having a relatively passive capacity for being rewarded by prediction and control to actively seeking it.

The human brain appears to be designed to notice and look for connections in perceived events and between new information and that already stored in memory. It is designed to detect regularities and patterns and to connect events that occur in sequence, making causal inferences under certain conditions (Dennis, 1991; Gelman & Kalish, 1993; Sylwester, 1995). Children also form categories spontaneously (Gelman, 1998), suggesting an innate tendency to classify information according to perceived similarities (Karmiloff-Smith, 1993). The brain appears to search for "meaning" (Changeux & Dehaene, 1993).

Models of Executive Functioning and Motivation

Annette Karmiloff-Smith (1993) believes that the child's brain spontaneously organizes itself. She proposes three assumptions that are needed to support this "constructivist" view of the child's organizational capacities. The first assumption is that the brain has some "innately specified information that allows it to attend to persons, objects, space, cause–effect relations, number, language, and so forth that channels the way in which it computes these representations. . . . These predispositions do not preclude the need for subsequent learning, but they constrain what is subsequently learned." Her second assumption is that the brain has a "number of innately specified processes" that support self-organization. These processes include "mechanisms for inferential processes, for deductive reasoning and for hypothesis testing." Finally, she assumes that the brain is "set to begin exploring and representing [the environment] from birth," is motivated to "try" to (mentally) organize the environment, and is also motivated to try to organize its own internal representations (p. 595). The environment acts as a "trigger" for this organization and provides feedback that helps the child modify both behavior and mental representations.

Karmiloff-Smith believes that the "linguistic statements of others" provide one source of feedback, but that some organizing processes occur without external mediation (p. 596). (This position is more compatible with Piaget's theory than with Vygotsky's view of the sociocultural origins of higher-level thought.) She proposes more generally that the brain is designed to be curious and to organize information in ways that create meaning. Infants have innate capability and motivation for organization and do it spontaneously from birth. Older children and adults spontaneously experiment with different representations of a problem or situation—testing, elaborating, and improving their current mental models—even when this is not required by external demands or constraints.

Barkley (1997) has suggested that the executive functions of the human brain create an "instinct for self-control." He proposes that the capacity for self-regulation "is not taught but emerges as a result of an interaction between the child's maturing neurological capabilities for self-regulation (the executive functions) and his or her interactions with a social environment that stimulates, encourages, and places a premium on such behavior" (p. 227). The child is born with the capacity to develop (with age and experience) (1) self-regulated inhibitory processes, (2) a working memory that can remember, revise and plan activities, (3) internalized language that supports thinking and self-regulation, (4) a self-regulated motivational appraisal system, and (5) a behavior analysis and synthesis system that can covertly rehearse, revise, and reorganize behaviors for more effective functioning. According to Barkley, these executive capacities are primarily "instinctive," in the sense of being coded in the genes, and are supported by the prefrontal cortex of the brain. The social environment nourishes and channels, but does not create them. This proposal challenges Vygotsky's view of the social and linguistic origins of self-regulation.

Emotions, Motivation, and Self-Regulation

Emotional responses exert powerful influences on self-regulation. They drive attention and form the basis for motivation and goal selection. Some emotional reactions appear to have evolved with behavioral responses as part of the human adaptive system for survival. Damasio (1984) differentiates between these "primary" reactions and "secondary" emotions. He suggests that primary emotional reactions, such as startle/fear responses to loud noises or falling, are innate and are likely to be triggered automatically. Secondary emotions, such as fear of doing badly on tests or pleasure at seeing a friend, are learned and are easier to control.

The principal brain structures that mediate emotional reactions are in the limbic system, a middle area of the brain between the brain stem and the cerebral cortex. The limbic system is especially important in (innate) primary emotional reactions. Specialized areas in the right cerebral hemisphere and the frontal lobes are more involved in (learned) secondary emotional responses that are cognitively mediated. There are more neural fibers connecting the limbic system to the logical and rational centers in the cerebral cortex than traveling in the opposite direction, so emotions are more likely to influence thinking and decision making than rational processes are to change emotions (Sylwester, 1995). This suggests that it is easier for people to control the expression of emotions than to change the way they really feel.

Most incoming information is sent to the sensory and frontal lobes for analysis, but emotion-laden information can be sent directly to a structure called the amygdala in the limbic system, bypassing more conscious and rational analyses. This allows quick responses to potential dangers but makes the responses less accessible for voluntary control. Because primary emotional reactions tend to bypass conscious and rational processing centers, situations that induce feelings of danger or threat reduce an individual's capacity for self-regulation in such circumstances. A child who is afraid of failure may be less able to mobilize her executive functions to achieve success in problem solving. A child who is afraid of rejection or bullying may be less able to reorganize behaviors to try to be more accepted and successful in social situations.

Internal or "intrinsic" motivators induce feelings of self-direction and control, and external or extrinsic motivators can induce stress and feelings of loss of control (Gazzaniga, 1985, 1992; Seligman, 1991). External rewards and punishments may not only undermine intrinsic motivation (Deci & Ryan, 1985, 1987), they may also reduce a child's capacity for self-regulation by arousing emotional responses that limit higher level thinking and flexible executive functioning. Moreover, attention may be focused on reinforcement and punishment contingencies, rather than on analyzing complex cues and problem-solving strategies. Rather than use executive capacities to reflect upon, play with, experiment with, and improve plans and strategies, the child may set a goal of obtaining a reward or avoiding a punishment. The intrinsic goals of the executive system appear to be (1) to organize information so it is understandable or "meaningful," (2) to be able to anticipate events, and (3) to find a *better* or *more interesting* way to solve a problem or reach a goal—including the goal of self-regulation itself (Barkley, 1997).

CONTROLLING EMOTIONS AND BEHAVIOR

The systems controlling behavioral inhibition and nonverbal working memory provide the infant's earliest executive control (Barkley, 1997). Although there are individual differences, the capacity to delay a response and mentally represent visual information during the delay appears to be present as early as 5 to 12 months (Hofstadter & Resnick, 1996). Self-regulation of arousal and emotion (affect) also appears to begin very early in the first year of life (Kopp, 1989, 1992).

Regulation of Emotions

Kopp (1989) has suggested that a rudimentary form of emotion regulation can be observed in 3- to 9-month-old infants. For instance, they turn away from sources of unpleasant arousal to soothe themselves. Toward the end of the first year they use self-distraction, such as attending to pleasurable toys, or self-soothing movements, such as sucking on body parts. Between 12 and 18 months they learn to move away from sources of distress and to gain caregiver help in reducing negative emotional states. By the second or third year, Kopp proposes, children are aware enough to understand that they not only feel emotions but can also cope with them themselves to some degree. They can often identify the source of their distress and can use a variety of strategies to reduce or cope with it. They may comfort themselves with a transitional object (a loved toy or blanket), seek help from an adult, or attempt to negotiate with another person.

Sroufe (1995) suggests that different experiences, particularly with caregivers, can lead to differences in the brain circuits that mediate emotions and can result in "variations in the autoregulation of affect and self-regulation more generally" (p. 203). In support of this view there is evidence that socialization experiences can produce neurohormonal changes in the developing brain (Schore, 1994). Warm, responsive care in infancy appears to protect children to some degree against the negative effects of later stress and the hormone cortisol, which can make the brain more vulnerable to processes that destroy neurons and reduce the number of connections between neurons (Gunnar, 1996). The responsiveness of the mother or primary caregiver to the infant's biological rhythms and behavioral signals also appears to help the infant regulate her own biological and emotional systems (Hofer, 1995).

The development of language marks an important milestone in executive control, but a child has begun to regulate emotional states before she uses language (Kopp, 1989). According to Barkley (1997), the child has begun to develop three components of self-regulation before speech develops: (1) behavioral inhibition, (2) nonverbal (representational) working memory, and (3) self-regulation of emotion and arousal states. Language, whether used for communication with others or for the self in private speech, becomes increasingly powerful as a means of interpreting and controlling emotional expression.

A child begins to talk about her emotions between 18 and 30 months. She may also begin to use language to try to bargain with another child who has taken her toy or with an adult who is constraining her. By school age she can use verbal as well as physical strategies to cope with frustration (Mischel & Mischel, 1983; Mischel, Shoda, & Rodriguez, 1989).

Regulation of Behavior

Behavioral inhibition is an executive process with a central role in self-regulation. In Barkley's (1997) model, it is a prerequisite for all other executive functioning. He suggests that in order to regulate behavior a child must be capable of the three interrelated processes: (1) inhibiting initial ("prepotent") responses to an event, (2) stopping ongoing responses, and (3) controlling interference with ongoing activities. Inhibition "permits, supports, and protects the executive functions" by providing the delay necessary for decisions and self-directed actions to occur (p. 51). Inhibitory controls increase markedly between the ages of 2 and 3 (Masters & Binger, 1978).

Before the age of 3, children's capacity to follow rules given by caregivers is present but not well developed (Barkley, 1997; Kopp, 1982; Luria, 1961). Before this age children follow instructions to start a behavior better than instructions to refrain from or stop a behavior (Luria, 1961). In addition, they tend not to stick to rules in sorting activities or games (Zelazo, Resnick, & Pinon, 1995). Because reminders do not improve the child's performance, the shift in capacity to follow rules of behavior after age 3 appears to have more to do with the ability to inhibit responses than to remembering the rules (Zelazo et al., 1995).

The prefrontal cortex is involved in inhibiting responses (Cummings, 1995) and in working memory (Fuster, 1989; Goldman-Rakic, 1995). It is also involved when an individual must decide what to do (Passingham, 1993). When a task is being learned and controlled decisions about behavior must be made, the prefrontal cortex is activated. Later, if the task can be executed automatically, the prefrontal cortex is not engaged. The executive functions in this area of the brain are involved when behavior involves voluntary action and choice. Brain imaging studies have revealed a large increase in metabolic rates (Chugani, Phelps, & Mazziotta, 1993) and in the development of connections between neurons (Huttenlocher, 1993) in the prefrontal cortex between the ages of 2 and 4 years.

Private speech is observable in children by the time they are 3 to 5 years old. It becomes increasingly covert during the early elementary years and appears to be completely internalized by the 9th to 12th years (Berk, 1992). Private speech also appears to be increasingly powerful in controlling behavior. It supports increased delay of gratification (Mischel et al., 1989) and self-control (Kopp, 1982). It functions as a means of self-guidance (Luria, 1961) and problem solving (Berk, 1992). Barkley (1997) suggests that private speech replaces nonverbal representation as the basis for working memory and supports complex rule-governed behavior. He notes that "by the time that rules given by others are coming to exert some control over behavior, speech is becoming turned on the self as a means of self-control" (p. 215). In addition to helping children control their behavior independently, private speech facilitates the development of self-motivation and emotional self-regulation. It allows "the separation of affect from events and one's initial reaction to them" so that the child can develop perspective and objectivity (p. 226).

CONTROLLING COGNITIVE PROCESSES

Over the course of their development, children acquire richer and more complex cognitive systems and gain more sophisticated control over their thinking and learning. Research has documented an increasing ability to detect patterns (Farnham-Diggory, 1992; Gibson, 1969), increasingly complex working memory programs (Case, 1985, 1992), increasingly complex rules and strategies (Siegler, 1986, 1989), an increasing ability to plan (Brown & DeLoach, 1978; Das, 1984; Friedman et al., 1987) and increasing metacognitive abilities (Flavell, 1978, 1993; Sternberg, 1984). Development in each of these areas supports the child's growing self-regulatory capacities. In addition to increases in cognitive ability, Karmiloff-Smith (1979, 1993) suggests a growing "quest for (cognitive) control" that provides intrinsic motivation for cognitive self-regulation.

Brain development as well as experience supports the development of this control. Psychological changes in the frontal lobes in the second half of the first year parallel the cognitive changes in infants suggested by Piaget (A. Diamond, 1993; Goldman-Rakic, 1993). There are also important advances in frontal lobe functioning at ages 6 and 10 and in late adolescence that parallel advances in executive control (Welsh, Pennington, & Groisser, 1991). Generally, the expansion of frontal lobe areas "from the lowest mammals up to man parallels the development of cognition" (Changeux & Dehaune, 1993, p. 369).

Although frontal lobe development is not complete until adulthood, certain behavioral competencies such as selective attention and inhibition emerge during the first year of life (Denckla & Reader, 1993). Barkley (1997) notes that most of the executive functions described in his "hybrid" model are well under way by the early school years and that there is a marked increase in self-regulation between the ages of 5 and 7. Progressive increases in the power to inhibit and control behavior are associated with "an increase in the various forms of working memory" that allows the child to "hold events online and even manipulate them" (p. 224). In early development this capacity allows the child to imitate behavior, especially complex, novel sequences of behavior. Even nonverbal working memory provides "a mental window on time" through which "hindsight . . . and forethought can develop" (p. 224). It allows a child to anticipate and begin preparations for future events and leads to a "psychological sense of time" (p. 225).

Goldman-Rakic (1987) proposes that the frontal cortex is essentially a working memory system in which associations are formed between goals, environmental stimuli, and stored knowledge. Baddeley (1986; Baddeley, Della Salla, Gray, Papagno, & Spinnler, 1997) defines working memory as a system for the temporary maintenance and manipulation of information. He notes that by far the most complex of the components of working memory is the "central executive, which is thought to act as a general attentional resource and to be involved in reasoning, decision making, calculation, comprehension and long-term as well as short-term memory" (Baddeley et al., 1997, pp. 64–65). Kopp (1982) suggests that self-awareness emerges with the progressive development of working memory.

The most forward part of the frontal cortex, the prefrontal areas, are generally considered to account for reasoning (Goldman-Rakic, 1987; Stuss & Benson, 1986), intentionality (Changeux & Dehaene, 1993), and planning (Shallice, 1988). Damage (or lesions) in these areas interferes with forming and carrying out plans and anticipating consequences. Individuals with frontal lobe impairments grasp and use any object presented to them "as if they had become dependent upon sensory stimulation" for action (Changeux & Dehaene, 1993, p. 369). The prefrontal cortex appears to have a "*prospective* function in anticipating and planning and a *retrospective* one in maintaining it in a provisional memory until the goal is reached" (Changeux & Dehaene, 1993, p. 390).

In an overview of developmental changes Barkley (1997) proposes that as the executive processes develop, the control of behavior "shifts from being context-dependent and contingency-shaped (externally governed) to being increasingly regulated by internally represented information" (p. 225). There is a decreasing need for "immediate and frequent" external reinforcers and an increasing ability to deal with delayed rewards and goals. Private speech provides another means of mentally representing information that expands the child's "repertoire for rule-governed behavior" and assists in shifting control over behavior from the environment to the child. He notes that children's private speech "seems less designed to control their immediate behavior than to improve later performance of similar tasks through verbal problem-solving, such as self-questioning, problem clarification, and conjecturing about possible rules" (p. 215).

Norman and Shallice (1986; Shallice, 1988) focus on flexibility and focus in their model of executive functioning. They contend that cognitive activities are controlled in one of two ways:

1. Most mental operations are routine and are run off automatically by the brain. Responses are triggered by environmental cues that evoke specific schemas or sets of responses with many subcomponents. The priority of one response over another is determined by "contention scheduling," where the relative importance of different actions is evaluated and routine behaviors are adjusted accordingly.
2. When automatic, routine operations are inappropriate, inadequate, or nonexistent (because a situation is changed or challenging or novel) a "Supervisory Activity System" (SAS) is activated. This system allows deliberate voluntary decisions. When the SAS is impaired, the individual may respond with rigid, inflexible (perseverative) behavior, or with inappropri-

ate behavior. She may have difficulty in changing responses or may not be able to inhibit irrelevant responses to random distracting cues.

Others have also suggested that as executive functions improve, distraction and task-irrelevant activities decrease and goal-directed persistence increases (Barkley, 1997; Posner & Presti, 1987). Improved executive functions allow the child to carry out tasks more effectively and efficiently. According to Barkley's (1997) model, increases in the ability to "reconstitute" behavior contribute to both greater flexibility of responding and greater efficiency in task accomplishment. Unnecessary behavioral components are evaluated and discarded, and more efficient strategies are increasingly deployed. If goal-directed actions are interrupted, children demonstrate a growing ability to resist distraction or to return to ongoing activities after interruptions. "A sense of time, timing, and timeliness in behavior should be progressively more evident across development as the capacity to organize behavior across time grows" (p. 227).

ENVIRONMENTAL EFFECTS ON THE DEVELOPMENT OF CONTROL SYSTEMS IN THE BRAIN

An increasing amount of research is documenting the importance of the environment, and children's experiences in the environment, to the development of their brains. Shore (1997) has reviewed what has been learned about brain development and experience in several major areas. It is now clear that (1) development involves an "interplay" or interaction between nature and nurture, (2) the brain is more plastic during certain sensitive periods of development, so the timing of positive or negative influences is important, (3) early care is important, and (4) early intervention can influence development.

Nature Interacts with Nurture

Brain development is affected by environmental conditions before birth and throughout a child's development. The nourishment, environmental surroundings, care, and stimulation the child receives affects how the brain develops, how its neurons are connected, and

even its chemical balance. Children are born with different temperaments and genetic predispositions, but physical, social, emotional,
and cognitive aspects of the environment have an influence on which
connections in the brain survive. Studies of brain development are
helping to resolve controversy among psychological theories about
the relative importance of nature and nurture.

Changeux and Dehaene (1993) have integrated a large body of
information on neural development and proposed a neural model of
how the environment affects brain development. They argue that the
developing brain is not a tabula rasa. Its architecture is neither undif-
ferentiated (all the result of learning) nor preformed (all innate), but
is flexible within genetically determined constraints—especially in
the early stages of development. The brain comes equipped with
"multiple functional levels of organization" with, for instance, a
number of built-in ways of representing the visual and auditory
world.* These protorepresentations contain distinct characteristics
that help the brain "construct categories in an unlabeled world" (p.
367). They are "heavily interconnected via feedback loops, or
reentrant mechanisms, that make possible high-order regulations between levels" and are "cognitively penetrable" or influencable at
some stage of development.

There are certain periods when different evolving neural systems
are more sensitive to environmental influences. This produces a "limited randomness" or "fuzziness" in the developing systems that not
only "makes a final tuning of the connectivity necessary, but also offers the opportunity for an adaptive shaping" (p. 375). The systems
also act as "internal generators of variations, continuously anticipating and testing the outside world" with reference to the representations they are producing (p. 371). The developing brain is not only a
passive responder to external stimuli, but actively generates representations of the environment and actively tests evolving neural structures and systems against incoming information.

For developing brain areas the periods of greatest sensitivity to

---

*Changeux and Dehaene note the difference between the ways in which cognitive psychol-
ogists and neuroscientists define representation. Psychologists use representation to refer
to the structure of internalized information or to its content. In neuroscience the term refers to the "projection of sensory neurons onto defined areas of the brain, or the mappings
of given domains of the brain upon others" (p. 380).

environmental influences occurs during their periods of "maximal connectivity," when neuronal growth and density are at their height. The timing is different for different areas of the brain because they grow at different rates and reach maximum density at different ages. Periods of maximum sensitivity generally occur during the first 2 to 3 years of life, with increased plasticity remaining over the first decade or so while brain density is still elevated over adult levels and active pruning is still occurring.

During the periods of maximum variability there is a "competition" among developing systems. A "selection of synapses" takes place during these sensitive periods, followed by a "drastic elimination of connections" that are not activated. In a form of "neural Darwinism" (Edelman, 1987), connections are strengthened and preserved when they are used (thus showing their usefulness in adapting to the environment) and pruned out when they are not used. According to the Changeux and Dehaene model, "the effect of experience is intertwined with innate processes from development through the adult stage. The formation of brain architecture is not independent of cognitive processes, but, rather, is deeply impregnated by them, starting from the early stages of postnatal development" (1993, p. 379).

The Importance of Timing

It is clear that the brain's plasticity peaks during certain periods of development and is greatest early in life. This means that the timing of positive or negative experiences is very important. The brain is more able to compensate for physical damage during the first decade, but early experience seems to be particularly important because it interacts with the brain's self-organization. It helps establish the basic map of connections on which later connections will build.

Positive Experiences

Under stimulating conditions, brain activity and metabolism increases and the cortex increases in size as more connections and support systems are formed (Huttonlocher, 1993). Experiences activate, and thus preserve and strengthen, connections that help the child adapt to the environment. Lack of stimulation leads to lower metabolism and slower growth in the brain and, later, a greater reduction (pruning) of connections already formed, through lack of use (Huttonlocher, 1993).

Stimulation is particularly critical for specific areas of the brain during their sensitive periods of development. Visual and auditory stimulation, for instance, is especially important during the 2nd and 3rd months, when the level of cortical activity rises in the sensory–motor areas (Shore, 1997). The frontal cortex shows increased metabolic activity at about the 8th month and reaches a maximum between 12 and 24 months. However, as noted earlier, this activity does not decline significantly until after age 7 and does not decline to adult levels until age 16 (Huttonlocher, 1993). This indicates a longer period of plasticity for the frontal areas, which support higher cognitive and executive self-regulatory functions, than for any other part of the brain. This area was the last to develop in evolution and is the last to mature in human development. The extended period of "immaturity" may be required because our species needs the most learning to survive, and the organization of our high level cognitive and metacognitive processes requires a long time and many experiences.

Negative Experiences

Plasticity also creates vulnerability. Creatures that are more "hardwired" are equipped to survive without needing as much environmental input as the human child does. They do not have the child's vulnerability to inadequate or negative environmental circumstances. Just as appropriate stimulation and positive experiences support and expand development during early sensitive periods, negative experiences may be particularly damaging at these times. Shore (1997) summarized research demonstrating that a variety of negative circumstances early in life—trauma and neglect, institutionalization, maternal depression, and poverty—have negative effects on brain development and behavior. Reviewing research on the impact of trauma and neglect, she notes that abuse either before or after birth "can interfere with development of subcortical and limbic areas of the brain, resulting in extreme anxiety, depression and or the inability to form healthy attachments to others. Adverse experiences throughout childhood can also impair cognitive abilities, resulting in processing and problem-solving styles that predispose an individual to respond with aggression or violence to stressful or frustrating situations" (p. 40).

Living in institutions such as orphanages and hospitals has long-lasting negative effects on babies and young children (Frank et al., 1996; Gunnar, 1966; Spitz, 1945). Under conditions of severe sensory and social deprivation infants' brains are smaller and less developed, they reach developmental milestones more slowly, and they even die at higher than normal rates. For these children, the lack of a relationship with (or attachment to) a particular caregiver appears to be especially important. The presence of attentive caregivers helps to reduce or reverse the damage (depending on the child's age), but the impact of social deprivation on social development appears to be more difficult to reverse than cognitive deficits (Sroufe, 1995).

Researchers have found that babies with depressed mothers show reduced brain activity, particularly in the left frontal cortex that regulates outwardly directed emotions, and have elevated heart rates and cortisol levels (indicators of stress) (Dawson, Hessl, & Frey, 1994). They are also less active, have shorter attention spans, and appear less motivated to master new tasks than babies of mothers who are not depressed. Depressed mothers are more likely to be unresponsive to their babies or to interact negatively and intrusively with them. They are also likely to express more negative emotions.

Poverty has been associated with many environmental risks, such as poor nutrition and inadequate medical care, unsafe living conditions, and exposure to stress and violence (Shore, 1997). It is also associated with a number of developmental problems in children. Even children who are healthy at birth tend to show declines in mental, motor, and socioemotional development when they live in poverty (Egeland et al., 1993; Sroufe, 1989, 1995). Their difficulties include problems in self-regulation—such as difficulty in regulating their emotions, cooperating with other children, and playing independently by the preschool age—and, later, behavior control problems and ADHD. Sroufe and his colleagues (Sroufe, 1995; Egeland et al., 1993; Urban, Carlson, Egeland, & Sroufe, 1991) relate these problems to the negative environmental conditions associated with poverty.

The Importance of Early Care

Responsive early care and the development of a secure attachment to caregivers appear to be particularly important for all forms of development. Children are "primed for learning" during the first few years, and research has documented the impact of early care and nurture on their ability to learn and to regulate their emotions (Shore, 1997; Sroufe, 1995). As noted earlier in this chapter and in Chapter 3, warm and responsive care appears to buffer children against the negative effects of stress by changing their brains' chemical response to it (Egeland et al., 1993; Gunnar, 1996; Perry, 1996). Secure attachments to caregivers seem to prepare children to be confident and independent learners with strong social skills (Ainsworth & Bell, 1974; Erickson, Korfmacher, & Egeland, 1992).

The work of Hofer (1988, 1995) provides a biological explanation for the importance of attachment. He suggests that mothers begin to regulate the fetus even before birth through "placental transfer." Biologically active substances that support fetal development are conveyed in this way, and the mother's daily activities begin to set her baby's daily rhythms and sleep–wake cycles. After birth, caregiver responsiveness and the nature and timing of physical contact act as "hidden regulators." Infants in orphanages or chaotic homes fail grow at expected rates, and premature babies who receive more tactile stimulation and consistent care develop faster (Als, Lawhon, McAnulty, Gibes-Grosman, & Blickman, 1994; Frank et al., 1996; Hofer, 1995).

As noted earlier (in Chapter 3) a lack of responsive care or separation from adult attachment figures is associated with reduced brain development and long-lasting cognitive and social problems, including a proneness to violence (Perry, 1996; Renken et al., 1989). In addition to buffering children against environmental stress, sensitive, nurturant care can ameliorate the problems of children who are either withdrawn, passive and depressed, or overactive and aggressive (Greenspan & Benderly, 1997).

The Effectiveness of Early Intervention

There is mounting evidence that well-designed environmental interventions can improve the current condition and future prospects of children with medical, cognitive, or social problems—even those with brain damage or mental retardation. Shore (1997) reviewed findings from a number of intervention projects designed to help preterm infants, children with neurological impairments, autistic children, and those growing up in poverty. In general, early, intensive, individualized programs that take advantage of the sensitive periods in brain development and modify the everyday environment by involving parents are most effective.

The results of a program designed for preterm infants (Als & Gilkerson, 1995) emphasize the importance of the environment for the development of self-regulation. Hospital personnel were trained to observe the behavior of every infant and to individualize the caregiving plan based on characteristics such as the infant's sleep–wake cycle and use of self-soothing strategies. Parents were often present and they, with other caregivers, provided frequent physical contact. In addition, an effort was made to have the same caregivers available when parents were not present because they would be better able to recognize infants' signals and respond to them consistently. Under these intervention conditions preterm infants showed improved patterns of brain functioning, particularly in the frontal lobe, which is involved in regulating an infant's state of arousal during the first few months of life.

Environmental conditions clearly seem to be involved in the development of self-regulatory functions in the brain from birth, and probably before birth through the placental transfer suggested by Hofer (1988, 1995). Experience interacts with innate systems to activate maturing neural connections and to select (by stimulation) the pathways that will survive. There appears to be a long "sensitive period" for the development of self-regulatory functions, but experiences during the early childhood years lay a critical foundation for later development.

SUMMARY

Research on the development of the human brain has increased dramatically in recent years. Findings from this research have focused attention on the importance of the early childhood period—particularly the first 3 years—in fostering this development. Plasticity is greatest during this period. During the early years the brain produces more connections than it needs, and those that are not used are eliminated. This creates both opportunities for learning in a variety of areas and vulnerability to impoverished or adverse environmental conditions.

The frontal lobes of the brain support a variety of self-regulatory or executive functions: the ability to inhibit behavioral responses, control distractions, regulate emotions, hold and analyze information in working memory, generate and manage internal motivation, and plan and sequence activities, generating novel combinations from among those held in working memory. The frontal lobes develop more slowly than the other brain systems and remain immature and flexible for longer periods. This allows more time to form the complicated interconnections—among neural structures in the frontal lobes and between these and structures in other parts of the brain—that support higher-level cognitive processes and voluntary self-regulation.

The executive systems in the frontal lobes appear to have their own intrinsic "motivation" to organize, categorize, and predict stimulus events in the environment. These systems also appear to have an "instinct for self-control" that emerges as the child discovers her own self-regulatory capacities and, in interaction with the social and physical environment, discovers her ability to influence other people and external objects. The child's intrinsic motivation for self-regulation, understanding, and control can be affected (nourished or damped) by the types of external constraints and controls provided by the environment.

The frontal lobes have many connections with the emotional centers of the brain in the limbic system. Self-regulation of arousal and emotional responses begins in the first few months of life. Children develop increasing control over the expression of their emotions and over their behavior during the preschool years. They become able to obey requests from others to engage in certain behaviors and inhibit others. They can obey requests to instigate behaviors before being able to obey prohibitions or commands to stop ongoing activities. The use of private speech appears to support children's self-control and their ability to engage in complex rule-governed behaviors.

Brain development, especially in the frontal lobes, supports the child's growing cognitive control—of attention, working memory, and problem-solving processes. The prefrontal areas, the most forward part of the frontal cortex, are generally considered to account for reasoning, intentionality, and planning. The internalization of private speech appears to expand the cognitive repertoire by assisting working memory and mediating the (metacognitive) ability to reflect on internal cognitive activities. It helps children (and adults) plan, guide, and monitor their activities in a variety of complex situations.

The environment plays an important role in the development of the brain and the executive control systems in the frontal lobes. The environment influences brain development before birth and throughout life, but neural systems are particularly vulnerable to environmental effects during periods of "maximal connectivity" when the density of neural connections are at their height and being "pruned." During these sensitive periods both positive and negative experiences have maximal effects. Responsive early care and infant attachment to adults appear to be especially critical. Interactions with others support the healthy development of emotional centers of the brain and the frontal areas that regulate emotions. Disorganized and stressful environments, such as those encountered by children living in poverty, reduce or impair brain development and the development of self-regulation. Children with problems associated with brain functioning can be helped by well-designed remedial interventions. Interventions are most effective when they occur early, are intensive and individualized, and involve parents.

Table 6.1 summarizes information on brain development and the environmental effects on the development of motivation for self-regulation, and self-regulated emotions, behavior, and cognition.

TABLE 6.1. Brain Development, the Development of Self-Regulation, and Effects of the Environment on This Development

Area of development	Brain development	Effects of the environment
Motivation for self-regulation	Intrinsic goals of the executive system: • to organize information so it is understandable and meaningful • to be able to anticipate events • to find a better or more interesting way to solve a problem or reach a goal	Lack of coherence and meaning may impede the expression of intrinsic goals Lack of opportunities for choice, control, and becoming more effective may impede the expression of intrinsic goals
Self-regulation of emotion	Emotions exert a powerful influence on self-regulatory functions such as decision making and choice of goals Self-regulation of arousal begins in the first year Some strategies to control the expression of emotions develop in the second to third year	Early interactions with caregivers lead to neurohormonal changes in the brain Warm, responsive care protects against the negative effects of stress Responsiveness to biological rhythms and signals helps infants regulate biological and emotional systems Some evidence that early intervention can remedy some of the effects of inadequate early care
Self-regulation of behavior	The ability to inhibit behaviors develops even before speech (can inhibit initial responses to an event) The ability to inhibit behavior increases markedly between ages 2 and 3, before age 3 children are not good at following rules (can follow instruction to start an activity better than instruction to stop an activity); at age 3 can both start and stop following instructions Between ages 2 and 4 large increase in metabolic rates in executive (prefrontal) area of the cortex, which controls decision making and voluntary action Toddlers are able to comply with simple requests; at ages 3 to 5 children can follow rules and comply with increasingly more complex directions and rules Child increasingly able to control interference with an ongoing activity and maintain focus (attention)	Negative experiences (trauma, neglect, institutionalization, maternal depression, poverty) have negative effects on brain development and control of behavior and hinder healthy attachment to others Negative experiences may predispose an individual to respond with aggression or violence to stress or frustration Some evidence that early intervention can remedy some of the effects of negative early experiences
Self-regulation of cognitive processes	The brain spontaneously organizes itself (forms categories, notices and begins to anticipate regularities, detects contingencies, and makes cause–effect inferences) Increases in frontal lobe functioning take place in the second half of the first year, at about age 6, and at about age 10 Children have a nonverbal memory before the development of speech Increases in working memory capacity (facilitated by speech) parallel increases in intentionality, decision making, reasoning, and consciousness The prefrontal cortex is involved in intentionality, anticipation, planning, monitoring, attention control, decision making, and consciousness	Some evidence that young children need warm, responsive care for normal brain development Children need appropriate levels of stimulation for normal brain development Children need coherent environments for the brain to organize itself effectively Some evidence that early intervention can remedy some of the effects of inadequate early environments

Part II

Research to Practice: Supporting Self-Regulation in Early Childhood

The preceding chapters reviewed evidence from theory and research on the nature of self-regulation, how it develops, and how the environment influences its development. In the following three chapters, information derived from these reviews is applied to practice. Each begins with a summary overview of the development of self-regulation and environmental influences on development in the age range under consideration, based on the weight of evidence from theory and research. The overview integrates material on the development of emotional and behavioral control, prosocial behavior, control of cognitive processing, and motivation for control, to give a picture of the *whole child's* self-regulatory functions at the particular age and how each is affected by the environment. Sections follow with suggestions for practice, addressing both environmental circumstances and caregiver or teacher behaviors that are likely to support the growth of self-regulation in different areas of development.

165

7

―――

Supporting Self-Regulation
in Infants and Toddlers

OVERVIEW OF DEVELOPMENTAL
AND ENVIRONMENTAL INFLUENCES

The reviews of theory and research presented in Part I make it clear that active self-regulation begins very early in the first year of life and that important milestones are reached during the first 3 years. It is also clear that motivational, social–emotional, and cognitive areas of self-regulatory functioning are interrelated in the early years. They develop in interaction with each other and with stimulation from the social and physical environment. The environment affects neurological development, which in turn affects motivation, social and emotional self-regulation, and cognitive control.

Neurological Development

The infant comes equipped with a brain primed to organize stimulation from the environment and to develop executive self-regulatory functions (see Chapter 6). The human brain is genetically designed to search for, discover, and impose order and meaning on experience. It spontaneously organizes itself in interaction with the environment and is innately rewarded by finding patterns, categories, and predictable cause–effect sequences. This innate capacity for developing organization and executive control carries its own motivation with it. Many psychologists have proposed that children have innate motivation for self-regulation in the form of "effectance," competence, and control or self-regulation (see Chapter 2).

The overabundance of connections produced in the brain during the first 3 years provides opportunities for growth in a number of areas and the capacity to adapt to a variety of environmental circumstances. Stimulation selects the neural connections that survive, and a growing number of established pathways and constraints evolve. This process reduces flexibility but increases efficiency. The brain becomes increasingly hard-wired to do the tasks the environment requires of it—to organize the information and solve the problems the environment has presented and to do this with increasing proficiency and speed. The brain learns to perform many tasks automatically, without having to use working memory or the conscious, voluntary executive systems at all (see Chapter 5).

The process of selecting connections and reducing the density of neural connections produced in the first few years of life takes a number of years. There is a significant reduction in flexibility after the first decade, and the early childhood period is a time of maximum flexibility. The frontal and prefrontal lobes of the brain, which support the self-regulatory functions of voluntary attention, decision making, planning, and action, have a longer period of development and vulnerability to the environment than other brain functions. Significant declines in density, which indicate increasing efficiency but decreasing flexibility, do not occur until about age 7. This provides a longer period during which the environment can exert a formative influence on executive functioning.

Importance of the Human and Physical Environment

The child's early human and physical environment has a major impact on the strength and direction of self-regulatory functions. It provides stimulation, in the form of experiences with people and objects, that supports brain growth and preserves the neural connections that are activated. It provides the regularities and patterns that the brain builds on in later development. An increasing body of research suggests that certain types of environmental influences can help (or hinder) development more powerfully when they occur at specific ages or sensitive periods in development.

Children do not have to learn to be rewarded by pattern, predictability, and control, but the environment strengthens the tendency to seek them by providing opportunities for children to experience these rewards. Recognition of regularities leads to expectancies for recurrence, and experiences of finding order and pattern increase motivation to search for and find them. The child's recognition of self-produced effects leads to active efforts to produce such effects, and experiences of successful control of the self and the environment increase motivation to exercise this control. The environment can also weaken innate interest in pattern and control by providing few chances to have these cognitively rewarding experiences or by actively discouraging the child's efforts (see Chapter 2).

The environment is especially important in the very early development of self-regulation. Chapter 3 presents evidence that infants and toddlers regulate themselves largely in reaction to external stimulation and control. These experiences provide patterns and scaffolds for the child's efforts. The young child is more dependent than older children on stimulation from caregivers and the immediate environment. The social environment, especially interactions with primary caregivers, is innately salient to the infant and is especially important in shaping early self-regulation. Both the social and physical environments provide the data the child uses to construct an understanding of the world's coherence, predictability, and controllability and to build expectations for the future. Gradually, as brain and motor capacities develop in interaction with experience, external environmental constraints are internally represented and incorporated into self-regulatory functions (see Chapter 5).

As noted earlier, the child's functioning is integrated. Cognitive, social–emotional, and motivational aspects of self-regulation are interrelated in both development and performance. Effective and appropriate regulation of emotions, behavior, and cognitive processes requires motivation, cognitive organization, and warm, predictable relationships with other people. Especially in the young child, no area of functioning is isolated from the others.

SUPPORTING SELF-REGULATION IN INFANTS

Social and Emotional Behavior

The environment begins to influence the development of self-regulation even before birth (Hofer, 1988). In the intrauterine environment the mother's sleep–wake cycles, her changes in activity level, and the chemical substances that cross the placenta influence the developing brain and begin to regulate the child's functioning. In addition to ingested chemical substances, psychological states such as stress may influence the developing child if they produce chemical changes in the mother that are transferred through the placenta.

After birth, both the physical environment and caregivers' interactions with the child influence the development of early self-regulation. The regulation of arousal begins in the first few months, and regulation of emotional reactions begins in the 3- to 9-month period. The order and regularities in the environment, including day and night cycles, feeding schedules, and the activity and response patterns of caregivers, are incorporated into the child's own regulatory functioning. The child uses self-soothing techniques such as looking away and sucking to regulate arousal and emotions (Kopp, 1989, 1992), and caregiver responses to an infant's sleep–wake cycles and behavioral signals appear to help the infant regulate biological rhythms and emotional reactions (Hofer, 1995). In addition, infants start to be able to inhibit certain automatic emotional and behavioral responses to internal or external stimulation and engage in voluntary activities (Barkley, 1997). They also begin to develop expectancies about the social world and themselves in relation to others.

Although infants spontaneously begin to organize information from the environment and attempt to control their own movements and the external events they can influence, these activities can be delayed in severely impoverished or chaotic social and physical environments (Carlson & Earls, 1998; Frank et al., 1996). The social environment is particularly important. Physical contact and sensitive social stimulation and responsiveness are important for early self-regulatory development (Als & Gilkerson, 1995). When caregivers do not make verbal and physical contact with the infant and respond to her signals, or when they interact and respond unpredictably, the child's budding efforts to engage with the environment and find pattern and meaning, as well as engage with others and form social bonds, may be delayed or impaired (Hofer, 1995; Frank et al., 1996).

The quality of social interactions in the first year is especially important in the development of emotional and behavioral control (Sroufe, 1995). Infants are innately attracted to and responsive to other people. Caregiver behaviors influence the child's ability to exercise self-regulatory control and to detect and master the rhythms and rules of social functioning. Caregivers who are responsive to the infant's cycles and signals help the child learn to regulate these cycles and recognize the power of social signals. When the social environment is responsive and predictable enough for the development of expectancies, the child feels secure. A warm and loving social environment also promotes the development of empathy and caring for others, which appear to be prerequisites for later prosocial behaviors (Robinson et al., 1994; Zahn-Waxler et al., 1979).

Infants: 0 to 3 Months

Young infants need warm, sensitive, and predictable interactions with a primary caregiver and a physical environment that is interesting, responsive, and includes regular routines that they can learn to recognize and expect. As infants begin to adjust their sleep–wake cycles and arousal levels to the rhythms in their environments, the environment should be relatively consistent over time. To help establish these rhythms, periods of play and stimulation can be timed so that the environment and interactions with caregivers are quieter at night and before nap periods. Regularity in the environment does not mean rigid schedules. A child's periods of arousal and feeding needs evolve during the early months, and she must also learn to adapt to the needs of the family. Some children seem to be temperamentally more adaptive than others, but schedules that are too unchanging may reduce a child's ability to be flexible when circumstances require it.

Regular, predictable patterns in the environment, as well as responsive care, may also help children develop emotional control. They may be less frantic when hungry, tired, or otherwise upset when they learn predictable routines, and that their signals will summon help. Gradually, they quiet at the sight of the caregiver or the initiation of a familiar soothing routine before food or other material

comfort actually arrives. Expectations of regular events and responses from others, as well as self-soothing strategies, may assist the
development of emotional regulation.

Social interactions also help the child to regulate social behavior
in ways that are appropriate for the social partners she encounters.
To the extent that these interactions mirror the requirements of success in the larger environment, they help prepare for the future. The
infant discovers the capacity to communicate with and influence others as she experiences exchanges in which others respond to her signals. Dependable caregiver responses and regular social and physical
routines, which the infant can come to anticipate, help develop response patterns that can become increasingly self-regulated. The
child first begins to recognize familiar sequences, then starts to anticipate the steps, prepare for them, and respond appropriately. Later,
as routines are internalized, she can gradually begin to initiate and
actively influence or control them.

Appropriate levels of social interaction and physical stimulation
vary from child to child. Although all infants require gentle handling
and a relatively quiet and predictable environment, some can toler-
ate, or may relish, more stimulation and novelty than others. Some
may even *require* more stimulation to attract their interest or establish responsive interactions. Part of responsive care is paying attention to individual differences and to the ways an individual child signals interest and over- or understimulation, as well as responding to
signals for hunger, fatigue, and other types of pleasure or distress.

The signals of young infants are often subtle, so careful observation is necessary to learn to decode their messages. Children also
change and develop during this period, with accompanying changes
in their needs and signals. Periods when the infant is awake and alert
slowly lengthen, and the child's interest in the environment becomes
more pronounced. As caregivers learn to detect and respond to their
unconscious behavioral signals, young infants begin to learn which
signals bring results and begin to produce clearer signs of their needs
and interests. They learn to *try to communicate*.

Responsive interactions can be initiated or sustained by imitating the infant's vocalizations (grunts and coos) and facial expressions
(smiling, yawning) as well as by talking. Babies prefer soft, high-
register voices with frequent repetitions of words spoken in lilting,
song-like rhythms. Imitating children's sounds and expressions helps

them to recognize the interactive, turn-taking aspect of communication and allows them to begin to initiate and control it. Infants may enjoy repetition, song-like rhythms in speech, and simple songs partly because these make it easier for them to distinguish sound patterns. Other simple routines such as "peekaboo" allow anticipation of steps in a sequence. Naming body parts and familiar objects in rituals of play ("I kiss your nose" [while doing it], "I kiss your toes" [while doing it], etc.) or caregiving ("Now I wash the face," "Now I wash the fingers," etc.) also support a beginning association between words and objects—between sounds and meaning.

Young infants coordinate vocalizing, looking, and body movements in face-to-face interactions with a caregiver and soon learn to both follow and lead to keep such exchanges going. They may even cry if a social interaction ends before they are ready. The young infant is clearly responsive to, and enjoys, age-appropriate social exchanges that are adjusted to her individual level of arousal and sensory capacity.

Infants: 4 to 12 Months

Infants of 4 to 12 months are developing more differentiated and organized systems of emotions and behavior during this period, and their internal control is expanding. They are developing more complex strategies for soothing themselves, including moving toward or away from caregivers. Particular caregivers are now important, and children may become anxious in the presence of strangers. With a growing awareness of others as individuals, who are different from each other and separate from themselves, older infants may show a strong preference for familiar people, especially the primary caregiver.

The child may now feel safer and more confident in the presence of well-known people, whose behaviors and interaction patterns she can predict and influence. Having had experiences of being provided for and helped by these caregivers in the past, she has learned how to communicate with them and summon help when needed. Young children also look to caregivers for cues about how to respond to novel people, situations, or objects (Baldwin & Moses, 1996; Mumme, Fernald, & Herrera, 1996). The presence of familiar and trusted others gives them support and some degree of control over the situation.

Very young children play best with a trusted person nearby, even when exploring independently. They can experiment with the sensory–motor, social, and object-exploration routines they have learned to carry out, and know how to get help if they run into trouble or encounter something they cannot handle.

With familiar people, older infants are now more actively social. Their voluntary activities include attempts to get attention and create social effects, and they are aware of approval and disapproval. They enjoy interactions with parents and siblings and being included in family activities. Older infants give increasingly clear signals to others, such as holding out their arms to be picked up and reaching toward out-of-reach items they want. They babble and play with language and sounds and may try to imitate sounds or say a word or two by the end of this period. During the second half of the first year children recognize their own names and may begin to point to named objects or carry out simple directions and requests. They relish social games and rituals such as peekaboo and bye-bye, which become prototypes for self-regulated routines.

The ability to follow directions or participate in a social ritual shows an advance in self-regulation. Children now have the mental and motor control to carry out simple sequences independently, on request, or in interaction with others. They may also show increased interest in self-direction by resisting some caregiver requests. They become more assertive in their desire for control of their own actions and their disapproval for interference in chosen activities. This assertiveness becomes much more pronounced during the second year.

As children show growing interest in initiating social interaction, the caregiver can nourish this advance in self-directed action by noticing their attempts to influence others and responding in appropriate ways. Sometimes a child may simply be communicating her interest in an ongoing independent activity, sometimes she may want caregiver participation in the activity, and sometimes she may want social attention or interaction. By careful observation the caregiver can learn to discriminate the child's goal and respond appropriately, which supports the child's efforts to communicate.

Caregivers can also support children's internalization of routines by participating in the ritual social activities children in this age range enjoy. A child may like to drop an object and have it picked up, for instance, or to give an object on request and have it given back.

She may like to play hiding games or other games involving simple repeated sequences. She may enjoy imitating uncomplicated movements, appropriate to her age and capabilities, or following simple directions. All of these activities help the child internalize ordered sequences of actions, which she can later do independently. Many of these activities also involve language and associating words with specific actions and routines. A variety of early language experiences, even in the first year of life, have been associated with cognitive achievements (Tomasello, 1996).

As children begin to show their interest in self-direction and control by resisting others, it is important for parents and other caregivers to understand that these situations provide opportunities for promoting self-regulation. Although assertiveness and resistance can be difficult to deal with, the child's ability to have an idea of what to do, and to resist interference, is the beginning of positive self-direction and persistence. If a child's resistance is interpreted sympathetically, as interest in controlling her own behavior rather than simply as defiance or negative behavior, oppositional behavior patterns are less likely to be established. If the child is guided firmly but gently and positively, and is allowed to experiment safely with "choice" where possible, she is more likely to begin to learn to make adaptive choices and to guide her own behavior effectively. A positive guidance approach to discipline becomes even more important in the toddler years when the push for independence strengthens.

Voluntary Prosocial Behavior

Interactions with others support not only the development of control over behavior and emotional expression, but feelings about others, internalized rules about how others should be treated, and strategies for dealing with them. They lay the foundation for future social or antisocial attitudes and behaviors. From the beginning, social experiences shape the child's social understanding and expectations. These evolve into beliefs about what "ought" to be and internalized rules of behavior.

Infants have an innate need for social contact and an innate interest in other people. They also have an innate tendency to respond to the emotional expressions of others, which becomes evident early in life. Young infants pay special attention to faces and seem to be aware of affection and warmth, or tension, communicated in the way they are held and touched. They respond positively to warm, affectionate care, become apathetic or distressed in its absence, and may become upset when they sense anxiety, tension, or anger in others. They also show signs of distress and may cry when they hear others cry.

The infant's sensitivity to the emotions of other people underlines the importance of the social environment in the first 12 months. The emotional climate surrounding a child, and the expectations it generates, have a major impact on developing self-regulation (Sroufe, 1995). It affects developing social goals and the behavioral strategies the toddler will use to try to reach them. When children have learned to expect warm, supportive interactions with others and have observed concern for the feelings and welfare of others in the social environment, they are more likely to begin to imitate and internalize these prosocial attitudes and behaviors during the toddler years. If they have experienced and observed neglect, unresponsiveness, or hostility, they will learn to expect this treatment and to adopt the same strategies in interactions with others (Perry, 1996; Sroufe, 1989).

Early Cognition

In the first year of life infants notice and begin to look for patterns and novelty in the environment. As their store of experiences increases, they begin to be able to hold nonverbal representations of sensory–motor activities, people, objects, and events in working memory (Barkley, 1997). They also begin to organize information from these experiences into innately based "categories" that represent information about people, objects, space, number, and language (among other things) in different ways (Karmiloff-Smith, 1993). They are aware of cause–effect contingencies and delight in producing effects as early as 3 or 4 months of age (Papousek, 1967, 1969; Piaget, 1952; Watson, 1966). Infants begin to control some of their sensory–motor activities during the first year (Brazelton, 1962; Piaget, 1952, 1954) and begin to engage in intentional, goal-directed activities between 8 and 12 months (Piaget, 1962).

Infants: 0 to 3 Months

Regularities in the environment support the infant's beginning cognitive organization of the environment as well as the development of emotional self-regulation. Social stimulation and interesting objects and events also increase arousal, helping to differentiate, enhance, and extend periods of wakefulness and sleep. These periods become more clearly delineated, and the infant becomes more alert during the wakeful parts of the cycle.

Interesting objects and events invite both attention and sensory investigation. There is a sharp rise in activity in the brain regions that control sensory–motor functions during the first 3 months (Chugani, 1997), suggesting that this is a sensitive period for providing visual and auditory stimulation (Shore, 1997). Learning to discriminate both familiarity and novelty in sensory information helps the infant develop focused attention and beginning expectations about the environment. Sensory stimulation provides information from the environment that is increasingly "represented," neurologically and psychologically, in the child's mind. Developing executive systems need stimulation and information that can be represented in working memory to begin active self-regulatory functions (Barkley, 1997).

The physical environment is important. It provides stimulation, goals, and corrective feedback for action and supports the development of "intentionality" (Bruner, 1970). When the environment is sterile and lacks opportunities for interesting sensory experiences, or is overstimulating or chaotic, the child's cognitive engagement with the environment and mental organization may be delayed (Carlson & Earls, 1998). A sterile environment contains few stimulus events around which an infant can organize cycles of arousal and sleep. When an infant does not discover interesting objects and events in the environment, she is less likely to attend to the environment and look for them. If an infant is confused or overwhelmed by overstimulation or chaos, she is less able to regulate her own responses and to focus and explore. When the environment contains no people, objects, or events that respond to the infant's activities, she is less likely to attempt control.

The appropriate amount of stimulation and the relative amounts of familiar versus novel information that are appropriate for an individual infant must be determined by observation. Some children are overwhelmed by or uninterested in objects or events that please others. More objects or events are not necessarily better. Providing materials appropriate to the infant's developmental age and demonstrated skills, accompanied by careful attention to her responses, is the best way to match the level of stimulation to the child (Bronson, 1995).

Infants: 4 to 12 Months

The development of cognitive organization and voluntary exploration and control of objects typically involves sensory–motor activities during the 4- to 12-month period. The child learns to sit alone and may creep, crawl, or walk. She gains better control of her hands, developing the ability to grasp objects between the thumb and fingers and to manipulate them in a variety of ways. She develops simple strategies or behavioral routines for exploring objects. Objects may be held in one hand or passed between hands. They may be shaken, banged, squeezed, or dropped. Food is also explored, and by the second half of the first year the child may want to feed herself. Voluntary experimentation strategies also include opening and shutting things (doors, drawers, lids, boxes), filling and emptying containers, and pushing, dragging, or pulling objects. Many hours are spent practicing these strategies and exploring what can be done with both muscles and objects. Motor movements and activities with toys are remembered and repeated over and over with many variations as the child gains increasing control.

The perceptual properties of objects are examined, with eyes, ears, mouth, hands, and feet. The child is interested in color, size, shape, weight, texture, sound, taste, smell, and all aspects of the world that can be explored with the senses. The conditions under which objects appear and disappear, and how objects fit together or inside each other, are particularly fascinating during this period. Even in the first year of life the infant explores the perceptual characteristics and behavior of objects. If the environment is not arranged so that the child can exercise motor and perceptual skills, these skills will not develop as quickly or effectively (Carlson & Earls, 1998).

The environment must support the child's developing interest in movement, manipulation, exploration, and control in a number of ways. It must provide stimulation, goals, and corrective feedback for actions. The child learns how far to reach, what grasp is effective, and what actions produce interesting effects in interaction with objects in the environment. She also learns to initiate and direct ongoing actions in order to reach goals. Opportunities to engage in these activities also help the child regulate her efforts with increasing success. Through trial and error and active experimentation, she gradually learns to control her movements, how to explore and influence objects, and how objects behave when manipulated (Piaget, 1952, 1954). Play materials that challenge the child to perceive and try new things (at an appropriate level of novelty for the particular individual) support the development of self-regulation because they require adapting exploration strategies to an expanded set of circumstances. Materials that allow the child to produce visual or auditory effects through her own actions support an awareness of voluntary control.

In addition to providing appropriate objects and activities for children, caregivers can monitor their ongoing engagement with them, noticing and nourishing apparent interests, supporting the child in overcoming difficulties, and responding to the child's signals or efforts to communicate. They can learn to understand when the child is interested in exploring independently and can protect this involvement from interruption so that focus is maintained. They can learn to detect when the child needs help and respond promptly to her efforts to obtain it. Caregivers can also provide help in ways that support continuing independent effort and initiative, using "scaffolding" and the minimum amount of help necessary to allow the child to continue on her own. Although children enjoy and learn from independent exploration, caregivers can sometimes extend their play by participation that enriches but does not take over the activity. An adult might, for instance, explore materials side by side with a child, quietly modeling a behavior that the child is capable of but has not yet used.

Language is also important during the first year. Children understand words before they can produce them, and a language-rich environment supports language development. It is important that caregivers talk to children frequently, at a level that is responsive to their individual interests, capacities, and current activity. It is not helpful, however, to interrupt a busy, focused child, in the midst of a concentrated exploration of materials, with a barrage of language that distracts her. Verbal accompaniment to social routines and talking about what is going on during caregiving and joint play activities help children associate words with specific objects, actions, people, and body parts.

Providing safe, child-proofed spaces that allow opportunities for the exercise of developing motor activity also becomes important as the child becomes mobile. Focused attention and voluntary action are nourished when a child can explore freely in an area prepared to be interesting, challenging, supportive, and safe for her developmental level. These prepared areas should grow larger as the child develops more mobility, and the materials and furnishings should evolve to reflect changing interests and skills.

Not all children respond in the same way, show interest in the same activities, or develop at the same speed. Individual differences in activity level and the tendency to interact with people and objects around them may especially affect the development of self-regulation during this period (Kopp, 1982). Some children are interested in more intense and fast-paced experiences while others prefer slower and gentler interactions with people and objects. Children also differ in their preference for novelty (Kagan, 1997). Caregivers can learn to recognize individual infants' reactions to people, situations, and objects and can modify their interaction styles and preparation of the environment to accommodate these differences. They can provide a more stimulating social and physical environment for an apathetic or inactive child, a soothing and predictable one for the child who is fearful or upset by novelty, and a calm, focused environment for a child who is highly active or distractible.

Motivation for Self-Regulation

From the earliest months of life, the environment can support a child's intrinsic capacity to be rewarded by prediction, effectance, and control. During this period the child needs to find pattern, predictability, and meaning (personal significance) in the environment and to find that she can be effective within it—in interactions with both people and objects. Experiences of this kind increase motivation to find order and pattern and to be effective and self-regulating. The child also needs to discover that she is valued and that others should be valued, which nourish motivation for prosocial behavior.

From early infancy, children are rewarded by being able to anticipate or predict events, to control their activities and to produce effects in the environment (Bruner, 1970; Piaget, 1952; White, 1959). A generalized motivation for competence and mastery evolves as children have positive and successful experiences in these areas, and they become increasingly active in seeking them. The infant also needs to find the environment interesting, with appropriate amounts of consistency for recognition and prediction, and novelty to challenge and extend the child's understanding. The caregiver's actions are particularly critical for this age group, because infants are so dependent on caregivers to provide appropriate experiences for them.

In order to foster recognition, people, objects and events have to recur frequently enough and be salient enough for the infant to remember them. Primary caregivers, for instance, may be recognized before other people because they are often present and because they engage the infant in emotionally rewarding or arousing situations, such as feeding, comforting, and active social interaction. A special bottle or toy may be recognized because it frequently appears and is associated with pleasurable arousal and satisfaction. It is also associated with a variety of sensory experiences—sight, touch, taste, sound, and motor movements—that provide stimulus cues for memory. Certain routines, such as feeding, bedtime, and simple social play rituals, are remembered because they occur frequently, in roughly the same sequence, and are interesting, comforting, arousing, or otherwise emotionally salient.

Some infants will notice regularities in their environments more quickly than others, so it is not possible to specify how frequently a person, object, or sequence of events must recur for recognition and (later) anticipation. Emotional arousal aids memory, but more is not always better. Optimal levels of arousal are best for learning; too little leads to boredom and too much to overstimulation or fear. However, "optimal" levels vary with individual temperament, previous experience, and state of arousal (Fiske & Maddi, 1961; Helson, 1964; Hunt, 1960).

Caregivers can modulate the intensity and tempo of an activity so that it is congruent with the child's state. A rested and alert infant may be ready for more novelty and stimulation than a slightly sleepy or hungry one. An infant's state may change frequently in the early months, so caregivers need to be alert and responsive. Supporting the infant's engagement in activities appropriate to her state of arousal also helps support developing self-regulation. The child can begin to develop a repertoire of activities that range from arousing to soothing that can eventually be initiated spontaneously and carried out independently.

Infants also begin to notice the effects of their own actions on objects during the early months of life (Papousek, 1967; Piaget, 1952; Rovee-Collier, 1989; Watson, 1966). Caregivers can assist this awareness by putting objects in the infant's range of vision or touch, and arranging circumstances so that the child's actions produce interesting effects. Later, as the infant becomes more active in engaging the environment, the caregiver can support motivation by providing materials that interest the child and are responsive to her manipulations. Facilitating the young infant's engagement in activities that provoke interest and lead to anticipation and effective action supports motivation to engage in these activities.

Table 7.1 summarizes the types of self-regulation that are developing during the first year and the major environmental influences that contribute to development.

SUPPORTING SELF-REGULATION IN TODDLERS

The period between 12 and 36 months marks a significant advance in the child's self-regulatory abilities. There is a clear increase in voluntary control between 12 and 24 months, and in voluntary self-regulation between 24 and 36 months (Kopp, 1982). Inhibitory controls in the brain increase markedly between 24 and 36 months (Masters & Binger, 1978). Neural density in the frontal lobes reaches a maximum between 12 and 24 months (signaling a period of maximum flexibility and opportunities for maximum environmental input) and does not decline significantly until after age 7. This extended opportunity for environmental tuning of executive regulatory processes emphasizes the importance of children's experiences during this and the whole early childhood period.

Motivation for self-direction and independence strengthens during the toddler years, and the strong push for control can make this a challenging time. There is a qualitative shift in assertiveness as children become capable of symbolic representation and language. They become more aware of themselves and what they want and may resist interference or external control, especially if it appears to challenge their

TABLE 7.1. Developmental Milestones of Self-Regulation in Infancy and Major Environmental Supports

Domain of development	Milestones	Role of adults	Role of environment
Social/ emotional behavior	Regulation of arousal and sleep–wake cycles Responsive interactions with others Attempts to influence others Begins to anticipate and participate in simple social routines	Being sensitive to the infant's signals and "state" or condition (fatigue, hunger, readiness to play) Being responsive to the infant's signals and social initiations Paying attention to individual differences in the need for regularity, novelty, stimulation, etc. Engaging in warm, positive interactions with the infant that involve physical contact and the use of language Participating in predictable sequences of caregiving, social, and play routines that the infant can learn and participate in	Contains a consistent primary caregiver Contains a reasonable amount of order and routine that the infant can recognize and come to anticipate Contains alternating periods of stimulation and quiet that assist the child in regulating arousal and sleep–wake cycles
Prosocial behavior	Responsiveness to emotional expressions of others	Conveying warmth, respect, and caring in interactions with the infant and with others in the infant's environment Protecting the infant and others in the infant's environment by sanctioning verbal or physical aggression	Siblings or others interact in gentle and appropriate ways with the infant
Cognitive self-regulation	Focuses attention on specific others, objects, and own activities (reaching, grasping, manipulating) Notices regularities and novelties in the social and physical environment Begins to anticipate or predict sequences Begins to initiate behavior sequences with people and objects Notices the effects of own actions	Providing coherent and appropriate sights, sounds, and objects for the infant to explore Providing interesting and predictable event sequences and routines for the infant to discover and learn to anticipate Associating words with specific objects, actions, and routines	Contains visual and auditory stimulation that the infant can distinguish and monitor or explore Contains coherent and predictable patterns, routines, and sequences

(continued)

TABLE 7.1 (*continued*)

Domain of development	Milestones	Role of adults	Role of environment
Motivation for self-regulation	Early voluntary behaviors (intentionality) Experiments with and practices own actions (reaching, grasping, manipulating, moving, standing, etc.) Manipulates and explores objects Attempts to create interesting effects on objects by own actions (shaking, banging, dropping, fitting together, etc.)	Providing opportunities and appropriate objects for the infant to explore and manipulate Designing the environment so the infant can experience "being the cause" of interesting sights and events Protecting the infant from interference when engaged in a focused activity Providing assistance in ways that preserve the infant's focus, goal, and independent action	Is safe for infant activity and exploration Is interesting to the infant, with appropriate levels of familiarity and novelty (for the individual infant) Contains cause–effect contingencies that the infant can come to anticipate and manipulate

growing interest in regulating themselves. Children are becoming capable of complying with external requests to initiate and (at a later age) inhibit physical actions, communications, and emotional expressions, but they also recognize *and use* the power to say no.

Toddlers are increasingly aware of social rules. Younger toddlers may demonstrate "shame" when they are caught in forbidden acts (Erikson, 1963); older toddlers may show "deviation anxiety" when they perform or are about to perform such acts (Hoffman, 1985). As they approach age 3, children become increasingly capable of holding themselves back from engaging in prohibited activities and abiding by rules. They are also more aware of others and may be distressed when others transgress (Stipek et al., 1992).

In addition to becoming capable of conforming to social rules, toddlers engage in a variety of prosocial behaviors. They may spontaneously help or share with others and demonstrate empathy during the second year (Rheingold, 1982; Zahn-Waxler et al., 1979). During the third year they have a more sophisticated understanding of others' feelings, how they might help or comfort them, and what others expect of them (Dunn, 1988).

As toddlers struggle to understand and influence the social and physical environment, they develop a passionate interest in order, repetition, and routine. As they are learning to classify and predict aspects of their environment, they do not want them to change. Children explore and control objects more and more deliberately during this period and become interested in goal-oriented mastery activities (Jennings, 1993). Children's memory and ability to represent past experiences improves over these 2 years (Kail, 1990), allowing a more deliberate approach to choosing goals and the means to reach them. Starting with a trial and error approach, they gradually acquire simple, self-regulated action strategies (stacking, sorting, matching, fitting together) that they can use in a variety of situations. They are increasingly able to monitor their progress toward a goal, correct mistakes, and experiment with new approaches (Bruner, 1972; DeLoach & Brown, 1987; Piaget, 1952, 1954). During the toddler period children are controlling their choices and problem-solving in action; they are not yet planning ahead in novel situations (DeLisi, 1987) unless the actions required are few and specifically modeled for the child (Bauer et al., 1999).

Language develops rapidly during this period and contributes to self-regulation in a variety of ways. It helps children organize and classify their environment (Brown, 1973; Nelson, 1979) and adds to the accuracy and efficiency of memory (Kopp, 1982). Language also helps children remember and internalize rules. During the toddler period the external language of caregivers is more effective in than private speech in producing self-control (Luria, 1961; Vygotsky, 1962). However, the child is learning to label ongoing activities, which prepares her for the use of private speech to guide behavior later.

The social responsiveness of caregivers and the methods of guidance they use are especially important during the challenging toddler years. The child's self-regulatory abilities are expanding rapidly, and the will to exercise control is expanding even faster. Caregiver responsiveness shapes the child's sense of self and expectations about others. During this period of growing autonomy, the security and trust generated by responsive care leads to a more cooperative attitude (Ainsworth & Bell, 1972; Sroufe, 1990). The child is eager to preserve the warm and rewarding relationship with adults and more apt to imitate and internalize adult behaviors and values (Sroufe, 1995).

Coercive external control may gain immediate compliance, but it undermines the development of internal self-regulation (Lepper, 1983). Strategies that emphasize individual control over behavior, offer limited appropriate options, use suggestions rather than commands whenever possible, and focus on explanations and reasoning (brief explanations and simple cause–effect reasoning for this age) rather than demands are most likely to lead to internal control (Hoffman, 1970b; Maccoby, 1980). Providing opportunities to make choices and decisions and attributing inner control to the child supports self-regulation, by increasing the child's awareness of the decision-making process, and voluntary internal control. She is also encouraged to attribute the power to regulate behavior to herself and to develop an internal "locus of control."

The development of prosocial attitudes and behaviors is supported by a somewhat similar approach. A major requirement is a warm and responsive relationship with parents or caregivers, because the social climate affects the child's feelings about other people. Providing clear rules and principles of behavior that include the consequences of behavior for others, modeling and demonstrations of conviction (belief in prosocial principles) by adults, and attributing prosocial qualities to the child are strategies that support the development of these types of attitudes and behaviors (Robinson et al., 1994).

Caregivers also play a central role in supporting autonomy and competence during the toddler years. The quality of their relationships with the child affects her self-confidence and tendency to explore the environment (Damon & Hart, 1988). They support motivation for cognitive control and mastery when they provide developmentally appropriate materials, foster autonomous play, demonstrate reinforcing rather than restrictive attitudes toward the child's independence and mastery attempts, and mediate effective language skills (Crockenberg et al., 1996; Nucci et al., 1996; White, 1972).

Cognitive self-regulation depends on the patterns, categories, routines, and rules that the child's brain has been able to construct or represent from the material presented in the environment. It is important that the child's world be structured in ways that allow the detection of these regularities, in order to support both cognitive organization and the child's expectation of being able to bring coherence to experience. There are individual differences in children's ability to cope with different levels of stimulation and complexity, so it is necessary for caregivers to adjust the environment to appropriate levels for the child or children in their care.

It is also important that the environment provide opportunities for the child to make an impact on it and to notice the effects of her actions. Growing interest in cause–effect relationships (Jennings, 1993; Piaget, 1954) and in being a cause (Hunt, 1965; White, 1959) are supported in a responsive social and physical environment. Environments can nourish self-direction and goal-orientation when they include opportunities for appropriate choice, people who respond to the child's signals and influence attempts, and objects that can be manipulated in interesting ways or reward exploration by producing interesting effects. Play materials that encourage mastery activities support the development of problem-solving skills and strategies (Bronson, 1995).

The toddler period is also the primary language-learning period, and the linguistic environment mediates this development. Environments rich in opportunities for the child to hear and use language in ways that are meaningful to her help develop the ability to use these cultural "tools." Language supports not only human communication but mental organization, memory, and self-regulation, so the language environment is very important. Language labels draw attention to certain aspects of the perceptual world and ignore others. They tell the child what is important. They specify the way the culture organizes experience and the functional relationships it recognizes. The child incorporates this information and uses it to interpret other information from the environment and to regulate emotions, behavior, and thinking. To the extent that the environment fails to provide linguistic tools that are available in the culture, it fails to support development.

Social and Emotional Behavior

Parents and caregivers can support the toddler's development of internal control of emotions and behavior in a number of ways: by their arrangement of the environment, by their style of interaction with the child, by the types of guidance strategies they use, and by the behaviors and attitudes they model.

An important way of nourishing the growth of inner control is to provide an environment in which the toddler can exercise it successfully. Such an environment provides appropriate levels of freedom and constraint. Too little guidance is as ineffective in promoting inner control as too much (Baumrind, 1971, 1973). A few firm and consistent guidelines structure the child's expectations and give meaning to choice. The environment should also provide a number of opportunities for the child to practice self-regulation and choice.

In the social area there should be age- and skill-appropriate opportunities for observation, imitation, social interaction, and participation in activities with others. Observation and supported interaction with peers can help children learn social skills. The social environment should offer opportunities to learn and exercise social skills without overstimulation or excessive frustration, which may overwhelm developing self-regulation. The child should be able to master most of the social and physical challenges it presents without very many experiences of losing control. Adults can be observant and available to step in to prevent or help children resolve difficulties—before tears and tantrums if possible. Conflicts between children can present opportunities for learning to notice and respect the feelings of others, and for beginning to learn problem-solving approaches to the difficulties presented by differing interests and goals (Piaget, 1965). With young and inexperienced children, however, adult mediation is often necessary to support advances in understanding and in conflict resolution skills (Arsenio & Cooperman, 1996; Lepper, 1983).

An adult's style of guidance is very important for the development of inner control. Responsive and affectionate interactions that respect the child's developing autonomy and sense of self, support growth in self-direction (Nucci et al., 1996). Collaborative problem-solving approaches are especially useful (Crockenberg et al., 1996). Caregiver interaction styles that belittle or overwhelm a child, or are erratic and unpredictable, make the child feel confused, angry, or helpless and undermine the development of inner control in social situations. Coercive control is counterproductive (Lepper, 1983). It may elicit short-term compliance but does not promote internalization of control. When the coercive controller is not present, the child may stop following the guidelines.

More effective strategies support the child's sense of control over her own behavior. Using suggestions rather than demands, offering to help or join a child in a requested activity or emphasizing the attractiveness of the requested activity, may help. The caregiver can also offer selected (appropriate) choices. For instance, a child can be given a few reasonable choices related to how her daily routines are carried out. Activities such as dressing, eating, bathing, and toilet training can become battlegrounds if the child is not treated with sensitive consideration and understanding, as well as gentle firmness. It is important to avoid engagement in power struggles with children, because initial compliance leads to future compliance and initial resistance leads to future resistance (Lepper, 1983). The goal is to work *with* the child to support developing self-control whenever possible, rather than oppose it.

Modeling a desired behavior rather than demanding it is another effective approach (Bandura, 1986). This strategy is useful because young children are interested in imitating others, particularly those they care about (Kagan, 1958), and because it allows the child to *choose* to engage in the desired behavior (Lepper, 1981). Imitating modeled behaviors is also an important means of acquiring new skills and routines, which can then be attempted independently. Internalized representations of observed behaviors can ultimately be used as models or standards for self-regulated activities (Bandura, 1978).

Voluntary Prosocial Behavior

Toddlers are in the process of developing a more advanced understanding of others and of social rules, and an increased ability to act on their understanding. They now show clear evidence of empathy and begin to try to help and comfort others actively (Dunn, 1988; Zahn-Waxler & Radke-Yarrow, 1982). They are also becoming aware of social rules. During the second year toddlers begin to show distress or anxiety when they perform, are about to perform, or others perform a forbidden behavior. They try to inhibit or correct forbidden actions, check the reactions of adults to evaluate behaviors, and demonstrate shame when caught in transgressions.

Toddlers also begin to demonstrate spontaneous prosocial behaviors. They may spontaneously share a toy (although they will not reliably share when asked) or offer to help in household tasks (although this may also indicate an interest in mastering these tasks). As they approach the third year, toddlers may also begin to engage in very simple cooperative pretend play with a well-known peer or sibling. This early cooperation is more likely in interactions with older children who support a toddler's attempts to engage in play or when the play partner is very familiar and joint interaction patterns are well established. During the third year children begin to be able to initiate simple joint activities and make a few suggestions about how to proceed. They are beginning to understand the feelings, goals, and intentions (the "minds") of others (Dunn, 1988).

The environment mediates toddlers' growing social understanding and their tendency to engage in prosocial activities. In addition to the empathetic caregiving and demonstrated concern for others that provide a nurturing "climate" for prosocial development, caregivers can now provide verbalized rules of behavior that stress the effects of behavior on others. Zahn-Waxler, Radke-Yarrow, and their colleagues (Zahn-Waxler & Radke-Yarrow, 1982; Zahn-Waxler et al., 1979, 1992) have shown the effectiveness of this focus on others and of the active involvement of the primary caregiver(s) in both modeling and verbally expressing strong prosocial feelings and convictions. With older children an emphasis on "justice" and reciprocity may convince the mind (contribute to a cognitive understanding) of the value of cooperative and "moral" interactions with others (Kohlberg, 1969), but with young children it is necessary to win the heart (encourage emotional commitment) to a concern for the welfare of others. This concern is further supported when the child comes to view it as an internal characteristic (like being a girl or liking ice cream) and to expect to behave in prosocial ways because caregivers have attributed prosocial qualities to her.

Early Cognition

During the toddler years, caregivers can support the development of self-regulated learning and problem-solving skills by providing opportunities for the child to explore, experiment, and master simple tasks and by facilitating their efforts. Children are increasingly active in their efforts to explore the environment during this period; they like to choose and direct their own activities. Caregivers can provide appropriate choices, protect and support active focus and engagement, and, when necessary, scaffold the child's efforts to carry out activities successfully.

Careful preparation of areas where the child may play and experiment with relative freedom and independence is especially helpful for growing autonomy. Toddlers need a safe, orderly (predictable), interesting, and appropriately challenging environment in which to try out and expand their developing skills and understandings about the world. Safety is an important consideration, not only because toddlers are inexperienced and have limited motor skills, but because they are so curious. They notice details, and may find an electrical outlet (with holes that invite exploration) as interesting as a pegboard toy. Stopping toddlers from engaging in unsafe or inappropriate activities is much more difficult than prevention and may have negative effects on developing autonomy. Toddlers can also move quickly from one activity to another and may get into trouble before a caregiver can reach them. Appropriate precautions both help to keep children safe and give them more freedom for self-directed activities.

Order and predictability in the environment continue to be important. These attributes support the development of cognitive organization, the ability to focus attention effectively, and the ability to engage in self-directed exploratory and mastery activities successfully. Children can exercise more control when they know where to find things, what comes next, and how to participate. In a disorganized or unpredictable environment, they may feel helpless or confused and will find it harder to learn to cope effectively. The order and routine in the environment should be predictable rather than rigid. Some flexibility and change can be interesting and can teach children to be adaptable, but the constancies must be detectable and predictable enough for them to feel secure and able to initiate and direct their own activities successfully.

Protecting children's lengthening periods of focused attention in independent activities supports their growing self-direction and persistence. It is helpful to avoid unnecessary interruptions or distractions when children are involved in exploratory or mastery activities. Careful observation can help the caregiver respect children's ongoing involvement whenever possible.

Caregivers can also support toddlers' cognitive self-regulation by including interesting and challenging objects and activities in the environment. Play materials and social activities that give them opportunities to create effects by their own actions, to go through several steps to reach a goal, and to explore the sensory properties of their world are both interesting and challenging to this age group. Materials with these characteristics promote self-directed exploratory and mastery play. Caregivers can sometimes initiate and model new activities, then use the child's interest as a guide for continuing them. The goal is to extend the child's repertoire while respecting her independent ideas and actions. Simple social games, dramatic play, and participation in goal-directed chores or other household activities can give children a sense of mastery in the social environment, as well as provide opportunities to develop cognitive learning skills.

As children's verbal skills increase, language is an increasingly effective and important way to support self-regulation. In addition to supporting communication and categorization, labeling cause–effect relationships ("It spills when you tip the cup," "Hold on tight so you don't fall," "Push harder to make it go in") makes the relationships salient in the child's mind. Problem-solving strategies can also be suggested. Simple phrases that identify strategies ("The big ones go on the bottom," "Find the red pieces first"), as well as modeled actions, provide additional ways to encode these strategies in memory for later voluntary use. Moreover, such phrases provide directions that the child can begin to give herself in private speech.

Motivation for Self-Regulation

Toddlers have abundant motivation to regulate themselves, but their lack of skill can lead to frustration. Channeling motivation for autonomy toward appropriate and achievable goals can be especially challenging. Safety and appropriate boundaries are major concerns, because toddler experiments in self-direction may often exceed the constraints of the situation or their own capacities. They may climb too high, want to explore the microwave oven, or be determined to take off all their clothes in the supermarket. Although children in this age range need constant monitoring, the play environment can be arranged so that they can experiment safely and relatively freely and the need to say no is reduced as much as possible.

Guidance strategies that emphasize choice and encourage cooperation support motivation for both self-regulation and positive social behavior. Being able to choose whether to wear the red or the blue socks may avoid a toddler's resistance to putting on any socks at all. Toddlers' expanding skills and awareness of the ability to make choices are exciting and rewarding to them, and they will balk if these appear to be threatened. When they experience a few firm but tactfully presented guidelines for behavior (appropriate for their age and experience), cooperative attitudes on the part of adults, and a warm, trusting relationship with caregivers, resistance is minimized and motivation for self-regulation is preserved. If children believe that caregivers support their autonomy, they are more likely to accept the constraints they require.

Providing positive guidance, rather than restriction, criticism, and correction, is critical for maintaining an atmosphere in which self-control and cooperation are encouraged. This approach will not eliminate all resistance, but it allows the toddler to feel that her interest in independence is appreciated, and can produce desirable outcomes much of the time. She can begin to look for these desirable outcomes and exercise opportunities for choice in increasingly appropriate and effective ways.

Caregivers can encourage socially appropriate choices by supporting the child's efforts to participate and cooperate with others. Toddlers' desire to participate may be difficult for adults and older children, who must deal with their lack of skill, but support for their efforts to be contributing members of the social group increases their interest and skill in doing so. As toddlers watch and try to imitate what they see around them, caregivers may sometimes be surprised when they see themselves in these highly literal mirrors. Spontaneous interest in imitation and the desire to do what others do can be powerful aids to socialization and positive control of behavior, but they can also lead to difficulties. Very young children may be just as motivated to imitate undesirable behaviors as desirable ones, especially since they often do not know which is which. Caregivers can be careful to model behaviors they would like toddlers to copy and avoid behaviors they do not want imitated, such as shouting at children who are themselves prohibited from shouting. Toddlers also imitate the behaviors of other children. Although the caregiver's response to other children's behavior influences the likelihood that it will be imitated, the very young child's ability to learn from the consequences of another's behavior is limited. The toddler may still go up the slide immediately after she has observed another child fall off and get hurt. Preventing or eliminating negative models is a safer strategy with this age group.

Sensitive structuring of object play can support the toddler's developing interest in mastery. Objects that are rewarding to manipulate, demonstrate interesting cause–effect relationships, and provide attractive goals that the toddler can achieve with effort invite mastery attempts and encourage mastery motivation. Children (and adults) of all ages are motivated to engage in activities that generate feelings of competence and efficacy (Bandura, 1997; White, 1959).

Play materials that are a good "match" for a child's interests and level of development support both learning and motivation (Hunt, 1960, 1961). Tasks that are too easy may not maintain interest, and tasks that are too hard are frustrating. Sometimes adult assistance and support are necessary for successful manipulation or problem solving when new materials are introduced that require strategies unfamiliar to the child. Caregivers can briefly demonstrate ways to use the materials, or they can provide support (scaffolding) for the child's independent efforts in an initial joint play session (Berk & Winsler, 1995). Motivation for exploration and mastery is preserved when adult assistance is suggestive rather than directive and when it supports the child's independent efforts rather than ignoring or overriding them. Assistance should be targeted and offered at the child's point of difficulty; the adult should not "take over" the task and require that the child do it the adult's way.

During the toddler years, developing independence and autonomy is a critical issue. It is important that children's interest in autonomy be supported, that their skill in independent action be encouraged, and that they come to view their efforts at control in a positive light. If the toddler's push for autonomy is met with censure and opposition, the child may reduce her control attempts or may adopt a negative and resistant stance toward those who oppose her will. From this perspective, a major goal for caregivers of this age group is to create a social and physical environment that supports both autonomy and positive self-control.

Table 7.2 summarizes the types of self-regulation that are developing during the toddler years and the major environmental influences that contribute to development.

SUMMARY

Infants are equipped with a brain primed to develop self-regulatory functions. The environment influences the strength and direction of

TABLE 7.2. Developmental Milestones of Self-Regulation in Toddlers and Major Environmental Supports

Domain of development	Milestones	Role of adults	Role of environment
Social/ emotional behavior	Increasing voluntary control and voluntary self-regulation Growing ability to comply with external requests Increasing assertiveness and desire for independent action	Modeling behaviors desired in toddlers Using responsive guidance techniques that • use language to assist self-control • emphasize individual control over behavior • offer limited alternatives • use suggestions rather than commands • explain reasons for desired behaviors, using simple cause–effect reasoning Supervising play with peers and helping to prevent or resolve conflicts Providing opportunities for beginning pretend play	Contains a reasonable amount of order and routine that the toddler can recognize and predict (toddlers like order and predictability) Provides appropriate levels of freedom and constraint (with a few firm and consistent guidelines) Contains appropriate opportunities for observation, imitation, social interaction, and participation in activities with others Contains opportunities for carefully supervised interactions with peers
Prosocial behavior	Increasing awareness of others and the feelings of others (empathy) Some spontaneous helping, sharing, and comforting behaviors Increasing awareness of social rules and sanctions Increasing ability to inhibit prohibited activities	Providing a few clear rules and principles that include the consequences of behaviors for others Expressing concern for the feelings of others Expressing a strong value for prosocial behavior Conveying positive expectations about the child and her behavior Attributing prosocial qualities to the child	Provides a climate of positive and caring social interactions with the toddler and among others the toddler sees regularly Minimizes the toddler's exposure to negative, aggressive, or antisocial behaviors by others or in the media

(*continued*)

TABLE 7.2 (*continued*)

Domain of development	Milestones	Role of adults	Role of environment
Cognitive self-regulation	Wants predictable routines and resists change Can choose among a limited number of alternatives Begins to engage in goal-directed mastery tasks Begins to notice and correct errors in goal-directed activities Uses an increasing number of strategies to reach goals Shows cognitive organization by matching, sorting, and classifying	Providing developmentally appropriate play materials that support children's efforts to • experiment and discover the properties of materials (such as water and sand) • organize information (sorting, matching, classifying) • experiment and structure materials (with "open-ended" materials like blocks and clay) • understand and follow sequences (with multistep mastery tasks) • monitor and correct errors (in tasks with clear goals, such as puzzles) Mediating effective language skills Using scaffolding to broaden children's understanding and provide assistance	Provides safe and interesting places for the toddler to play and explore Contains an appropriate range of materials and, in group settings, a sufficient amount of materials so toddlers can play with them as long as they are interested Contains space and opportunity for action and investigation with protected spaces for uninterrupted play
Motivation for self-regulation	More deliberate choice of goals and resistance to alternatives Growing interest in cause–effect relationships and in experimentation with objects Growing interest in goal-directed mastery tasks Growing persistence in the pursuit of goals	Fostering autonomous play Demonstrating reinforcing attitudes toward toddler's independence and mastery efforts Designing the environment for independence Protecting the child's focused involvement and independent action	Is safe for toddler activity and independent action Contains opportunities for the toddler to practice self-regulation and choice Contains appropriate levels of challenge for the toddler's level of ability and interest

self-regulation. During the first 3 years a foundation is laid for a child's later emotional, social, and cognitive regulation and for the motivation to regulate herself in these areas. During the first year infants begin to adapt arousal cycles and emotional responses to the environment, to engage in voluntary behaviors, to categorize aspects of the environment and form expectancies, and to be more actively motivated to engage in these activities. During the toddler years children actively push toward independence. They develop the ability to carry out external requests and feel anxious if they violate rules. They also engage in more active exploration, experimentation, and mastery activities with objects, use simple strategies in interaction with people and objects, and have increasing motivation to be effective and competent. They also develop language and the ability to use it to label their own activities, influence the activities of others, and communicate with them more effectively.

The social and physical environment is particularly important during these early years. Caregivers provide the responsive care necessary for all areas of development. They also provide the mix of novelty and regularity that allows infants and toddlers to mentally organize their world. Their responsiveness to children's early signals and more active later attempts to influence others affects children's skill in interaction, feelings of effectiveness, and motivation for self-regulation in social situations. Caregivers' provision of objects and other contingencies that children can influence by their own actions and learn to master helps them learn effective strategies for exploration, mastery, and control. It also increases children's motivation to engage in these activities.

The characteristics of the social and physical environment that support developing self-regulation are always related to the characteristics of individual children, such as innate tendencies or temperaments, and their current state or context. Some characteristics change or evolve with children's developmental age and experience. Infants need warm, responsive care, environments they can learn to categorize and predict, and experiences of being effective in their social and physical worlds. Toddlers need scope and appropriate challenges for their developing autonomy, guidelines that provide both support and appropriate direction for developing inner control, and caregivers whom they care about and can trust to help them regulate behavior appropriately and develop new strategies and skills.

8

———

Supporting Self-Regulation
in Preschool
and Kindergarten Children

OVERVIEW OF DEVELOPMENTAL
AND ENVIRONMENTAL INFLUENCES

In contrast to toddlers, who typically need substantial guidance and support from adults to maintain control, preschool and kindergarten children are increasingly capable of voluntary internal self-regulation. They are better able than younger children to control their behavior and the way they express emotions (see Chapter 3). As "executive" inhibitory and working memory functions develop, they are more capable of refraining from forbidden behaviors and can hold in mind and carry out increasingly complex directions. They are also learning to use language more effectively to influence others and to regulate their own behavior. During these years children are shifting from primarily external to primarily internal control, but the environment continues to play a critical role in the development of self-regulation. It provides opportunities to develop new strategies and to practice increasing self-regulatory control. It also provides constraints within which children must operate.

Preschool and kindergarten children are increasingly interested in their peers and in interacting successfully with them. They want to be able to influence others and to be accepted and liked. During this period children can learn interaction strategies that accomplish both of these goals. They are more able to interact cooperatively with both peers and adults and are more successful in influencing them. Some strategies that are successful with peers may not be acceptable to adults. The environment plays a crucial role in the types of strategies children develop to solve social problems and reach social goals. Although relationships with peers are becoming more important, relationships with adults have more significant effects on the continued growth of effective and appropriate control.

Children in this age range are also capable of more advanced prosocial attitudes and actions (see Chapter 4). They are internalizing standards for behavior that they can use to guide their own actions in the absence of adults. They can talk about mental states, such as thinking and believing, and are developing a more sophisticated understanding of other minds. They try out roles in dramatic play and are increasingly able to understand how others may feel. Prosocial tendencies in individual children are becoming more consistent across situations and more stable over time. Antisocial tendencies such as aggression are also becoming more consistent and much harder to change by the elementary school years.

Adults are models, resources, and guides for children's developing independence. The way they carry out these roles strongly influences how children learn to guide themselves. During the preschool and kindergarten years children are influenced by both adult behaviors and adults' expressed beliefs and values (see Chapters 3 and 4). Toddlers copy words and behaviors, but older children begin to form judgments and make decisions based on what they observe. They begin to internalize what they perceive to be the attitudes and values of adults, especially those to whom they are emotionally attached, as they internalize standards for their own behavior.

Early socialization and continuing parental guidance practices affect children's tendency to regulate behavior in prosocial or antisocial ways. In addition, peer groups, teachers, and cultural factors such as the media play an increasingly important role in children's social understanding and self-regulation. Investigators have found that schools and teachers often have positive effects on prosocial behavior, but there are mixed results with respect to peers and the media (see Chapter 4). Peer interaction can help children understand the perspectives of others, and peers can model positive behaviors; however, they can also model undesirable behaviors, and unsupervised peer interaction can have negative effects on the development of prosocial tendencies (see Chapter 3).

The effects of television are also well documented. Viewing programs that model violence and antisocial behavior is associated with increased aggression when children are younger and increased aggression and crime for the same individuals later in life. Viewing programs that model prosocial behavior is associated with increased prosocial behavior and greater self-control in young children (see Chapter 4).

Preschool and kindergarten children are making great strides toward achieving cognitive self-regulation (see Chapter 5). They are learning how to do an increasing variety of tasks and how to approach learning activities in general. They are acquiring cognitive strategies that not only help them think and solve particular problems, but help them begin to control their own learning. Three- to six-year-old children are developing executive skills that allow them to select goals and tasks appropriate to their levels of skill and to work persistently to reach these goals. In a widening range of tasks they are able to resist distraction, use appropriate and effective strategies, monitor their progress (correcting their approach or summoning help if needed), and ultimately reach goals successfully. At these ages children may not consciously plan what to do before beginning a task, but they are beginning to "plan in action."

The development of cognitive self-regulation is also highly influenced by the environment (see Chapter 5). The opportunities provided in the physical environment, the rules of engagement with this environment given to children, and the types of support provided by adults influence the development of children's ability to carry out cognitive activities independently. Environments with interesting, challenging materials and activities that children can explore and master provide opportunities for them to learn and practice skills. When children are given choices and are allowed to learn from the consequences of their choices, they learn to direct their activities more effectively. Adult assistance in the form of scaffolding can also help children make expanded use of existing skills and acquire new ones.

Certain kinds of language experiences are particularly useful for helping children develop cognitive self-regulation. Questions that help children generate their own solutions foster the development of independent problem solving skills (Casey & Lippman, 1991; Casey & Tucker, 1994). Suggestions or linguistic modeling that focus attention on relevant features of a problem, or provide needed strategies for problem solving, can also help (Meichenbaum, 1984; Schunk & Zimmerman, 1994). For this age group, it is particularly important that strategies be offered in context, as solutions to specific problems the child is engaged in trying to solve, rather than taught in the abstract (Pressley et al., 1990). Strategies presented in this way are more likely to be internalized for future use. They may be provided either by adults or by more experienced peers (Berk & Winsler, 1995).

During the preschool and kindergarten period, motivation for social, emotional, and cognitive self-regulation is increasing as skill and success in these areas grow. Children are moving from a primary interest in exploring the environment to a focus on reaching goals. At the younger end of this age range, children focus on the *process* of reaching goals and may change goals if the process leads them away from their original idea. By the time they are 5, children are interested in the *products* they produce and persist in trying to reach preselected goals. They are also beginning to evaluate their products in relation to internal or external standards. Motivation is reduced if they do not view themselves as capable of meeting these standards.

Motivation for self-regulation is aroused when children believe that they are responsible for their actions, that they are capable of controlling them, and that they have choices (see Chapter 2). These conditions are important motivators for self-control in all areas—emotional, social, and cognitive. Coherence in the environment is also important. Children (and adults) regulate themselves according to the requirements of the social and physical environment, available goals in the environment, and increasingly internalized standards for judging the adequacy of their efforts (Bandura, 1997). For children to develop a clear understanding of the requirements in their environment, unambiguous goals, and standards for behavior and achievement that they can internalize, they must be able to detect the opportunities and constraints within particular settings. In environments that are disorganized and unpredictable, children have difficulty discovering the choices they have and the regularities and rules they can use to guide themselves (Minuchin, 1971).

APPLICATIONS TO PRACTICE

The social and physical environment continues to have a major influence on the development of self-regulation during the preschool and kindergarten years. Suggestions for supporting development are offered in four areas: (1) self-regulation of social and emotional behavior, (2) prosocial behavior, (3) cognitive self-regulation, and (4) motivation for self-regulation.

Self-Regulation of Social and Emotional Behavior

As preschool and kindergarten children develop increasing internal control over their emotions and behavior, they can be expected to obey rules appropriate to their developmental age with growing consistency. Although they are able to do more and more things independently, they do not yet have the experience and the executive capacity to function without some degree of adult supervision. Caregivers can support and nourish this growing independence by the way they provide guidance for children and by the way they arrange the environment.

Guidance Strategies

When giving directions or rules for behavior, adults should include rationales so that children can understand that there are reasons for rules. When reasons are not provided, children may believe that rules are arbitrary or relate only to the wishes of individuals. Self-guidance may be hindered under these conditions, because guidelines that are not understood are harder (or impossible) to predict and are therefore less likely to be followed in the absence of particular rule givers or in different settings.

Adults can also help children understand the relationship between their own goals and the behavioral strategies they are using to reach them. Preschool and kindergarten children sometimes fail to control their emotional responses or other behaviors. Adult reactions are most helpful for developing self-regulation when they focus on problem solving and more appropriate alternative behaviors, rather than punishment or retribution. This allows children to begin to be aware of the reasons why they are behaving in certain ways, the probable consequences of these strategies, and alternate (more appropriate or effective) ways to reach their goals. Children can begin to be aware of making choices and being able to control their behavior proactively by choosing strategies, rather than simply controlling behavior reactively by inhibiting sanctioned activities.

Children in this age range are beginning to understand reciprocity. They can be helped to see the relationship between their own rights or welfare and that of another child or the group. They can also learn to differentiate between emotions and behavior and to understand, for instance, that feeling angry can be separated from what one does about it. Caregivers can suggest that children express angry feelings in words rather than in physical aggression.

To promote the development of self-regulation, the goal is not to train children to comply with externally imposed rules and consequences, but to help them develop inner control, with appropriate and adaptive internal guidelines or standards for self-evaluation.

Arranging the Environment

Caregivers can arrange the environment so that it helps children to be aware of their ability to control behavior and supports them in doing so. Environments can be designed so that responsibilities, opportunities (choices), expectations, and consequences are clear, as well as appropriate for the child's interests and developmental age. In addition, they can encourage appropriate independent action and initiative.

Materials children are allowed to use can be made accessible to them without the intervention of adults. In home and group settings, materials can be placed in areas that children can reach without help. Appropriate spaces for different types of activities can also be assigned. Designated areas and procedures for the use of messy materials, such as paint, clay, and sand, can protect the child's efforts by being designed to support such activities and by providing the ground rules for appropriate independent use.

Rules for joint use of materials can also be designed so that children understand what is expected and do not need adults to mediate disputes. For instance, rules can specify how many children are permitted in an area and how "turns" are to be assigned. These can be discussed with the children and their ideas consulted. This approach gives children reasons for rules and makes it apparent that rules protect as well as restrict them. If certain guidelines are not working, children can be involved in discussions exploring why this might be so and devising more effective approaches. This strategy helps children understand that rules help a community to regulate itself and shows the relationship between individual and community self-regulation. It also gives them a degree of control over, and responsibility for, the process that can increase their understanding of why and how guidelines (rules, laws) are designed by groups. In addition, it increases children's emotional investment in the rules designed by their own group.

Prosocial Behavior

Preschool and kindergarten children are more actively involved with their peers than infants and toddlers and are more aware of the intentions and feelings of others. They are cognitively more sophisticated and able to engage in increasingly complex role-play over these years. They are also internalizing social rules and norms of behavior (as they are able to understand them) and act according to these guidelines with increasing consistency. Children are beginning to understand what they *should* do, and by age 5 or so they can feel not only embarrassment or "shame" but "guilt" when they transgress (see Chapter 4).

This is a time when social interaction styles—including prosocial or antisocial dispositions—are being formed as children try with increasing cognitive awareness to detect and understand social rules and mores. Consistent tendencies to behave in prosocial or antisocial ways emerge during this period. Research studies described in Chapter 4 have found significant correlations among giving, cooperating, sharing, helping, and comforting behaviors in 3- to 6-year-old children and that children who act in these ways are considered socially competent by their teachers.

Research has also suggested that caregivers can increase children's prosocial dispositions by (1) the types of guidance strategies they use, (2) the behavior and attitudes they model, and (3) the kinds of activities they expect or require children to perform, and that (4) peer and (5) media influences are important. The following paragraphs offer suggestions for supporting prosocial dispositions in preschool and kindergarten children in each of these areas.

Guidance Strategies

Guidance strategies used with preschool and kindergarten children build on the strategies used in earlier years and the social "climate" children have experienced, continue to experience, and have come to expect. It is increasingly hard to change children's emotional patterns and cognitive expectations as they grow older, so early experiences are especially important. Close and caring family relationships that continue through the first 6 years of children's lives set the stage for prosocial attitudes and behaviors. When it is clear to a child that both she and others are valued and cared for, this value system is likely to be internalized and the child develops an internal motive of caring for others (Hoffman, 1983).

To encourage prosocial dispositions, caregivers should use inductive guidance strategies that connect behavior with its effects ("If you hit him, it will hurt and he will cry") and help the child understand what others may be feeling ("She is crying because she bumped her head," "He is sad because you took his truck"). Adults should also give reasons for social rules and emphasize the effects of violations on others ("We take turns on the swing so everyone gets a chance," "We walk when we are in line so nobody gets bumped or tripped"). Positive behaviors that redress accidental or intended injuries to others can also be suggested ("If you give the truck back, he will feel better"). Physical punishments should not be used, because they model aggression and threat as a solution to social problems.

Adults can also encourage cooperative interactions among children by helping them learn strategies that support independent cooperation (Katz & McClellan, 1997). They can learn to suggest sharing or taking turns when there are disputes over materials, as well as ways of negotiating trade-offs that benefit both parties. They can also learn cooperative ways of influencing others and keeping cooperative interaction going. Suggesting goals or rules for play ("Let's build a space ship," "We have to move as many spaces

as the dots on the dice show"), ways to distribute roles or resources ("You can be the space cadet, and I'll be the robot," "I'll
use the flashlight, and you can have the space helmet, OK?" "I'll
use the red markers this time, because you had them last time"),
and continuing steps for ongoing activities ("Now let's say the
space ship is coming back to earth," "It's time for the baby to go
to bed now") support cooperative interaction in pretend activities
or games.

Adult Modeling

The adage that actions speak louder than words is especially true for
young children, but what adults say is also important as children
grow older. Caregivers teach children by everything they do and say,
including some emotional responses (shown in facial expressions and
body language) that they may think are not communicated. By the
preschool years children usually know when a caregiver is impatient,
angry, worried, or afraid, as well as whether the adult is happy or
sad. They can also infer attitudes from behavior, but do not understand complex motives. If an adult appears to be angry with a child
or punishes her, child observers may infer that the target of these reactions is "bad" or that the adult does not like her. Adults can provide interpretations that help children understand ("I don't like to see
our toys get broken, and I'm sure Andy will be more careful next
time," "If we throw the blocks, someone may get hurt. Jane can
come back to the block area when she is ready to use the blocks for
building").

How caregivers interpret social situations makes an increasing
impression on children as they come to understand symbolic communication and internalize linguistically mediated concepts. An adult's
explanations, such as "She didn't mean to hurt you; she bumped into
you by accident," can help children separate action from intention
and begin to consider intention in their responses. Prosocial actions,
emotions, and explanations provided by the people to whom children are attached have powerful effects on them. Caring behaviors
that are accompanied by clear emotional commitment and explanation of the moral lesson ("We *must* help people who are in trouble,"
"We should always give everyone a turn who wants one") are especially effective (Zahn-Waxler et al., 1979).

Adult Expectations

Encouraging children to take responsibility for tasks that serve the family or classroom community also helps them to develop responsible attitudes. When adults expect children to contribute to the common good at their level of ability, they internalize these expectations. Adults can also attribute prosocial motives to children ("You were generous to let Timmy play with your car," "You were kind to help Beth pick up the crayons she dropped"), which helps them to attribute these motives to themselves and expect to behave in similar ways in the future. Cross-cultural studies have suggested that caring for younger children is particularly associated with these prosocial dispositions (Whiting & Whiting, 1975). In families with several children or in mixed-age groups, caregivers can encourage older children to help and support younger ones.

Peer Influences

As noted earlier in this chapter and in Chapter 4, peers can have a positive or negative influence on children's prosocial behaviors and attitudes. Children are more likely to share and help when they see other children doing so, but they are also more likely to engage in negative behaviors when they see peers doing such things. Modeled aggression is learned, especially when aggression brings rewards or is ignored by adults (Bandura et al., 1963). To minimize negative modeling, peer interaction can be monitored by caregivers, who can provide appropriate guidance and actively support cooperative and caring prosocial activities.

Media Influences

Adults can also monitor and screen young children's media contacts. They can restrict access to inappropriate television programs and video games. Although this requires vigilance and firm determination, exposing children to primarily positive models during this vulnerable period can lead to long-term benefits. Preschool and kindergarten children are internalizing values, and their social understanding is limited. They may not connect violent actions with the punishment or negative outcomes that occur 40 minutes later. They also tend to think in absolutes (right or wrong, good or bad) and cannot understand relative values. When caregivers believe certain media experiences are valuable but too complex, they can help clarify children's understanding by watching movies or television programs with them and explaining or interpreting the action according to the values they wish to communicate. Access to the Internet is beginning to present similar challenges to caregivers.

Cognitive Self-Regulation

Preschool and kindergarten children are developing the capacity to engage in a widening range of cognitive activities independently. They are also "learning how to learn." Although they are not usually able to describe how they make decisions or the strategies they use, children in this age range are using executive functions in their cognitive activities. They are increasingly able to choose activities or tasks appropriate to their own level of skill, use effective strategies to carry them out, monitor their progress, correct their approach or summon help when needed, and resist distraction until their "process" or "product" goal is reached. Adults can support the development of these cognitive self-regulatory skills by the way they (1) arrange the learning environment and (2) provide assistance or "scaffolding" when children need it.

Arranging the Environment

The development of cognitive self-regulation is facilitated by opportunities to engage in self-chosen and self-regulated tasks as well as tasks scaffolded by adults or more experienced peers. Children's ability to choose and direct their own activities is supported when they have opportunities to choose from among appropriate alternatives and learn from the consequences of their choices. An environment that provides a variety of materials that interest and challenge children, at an appropriate level of difficulty, encourages choice. Adults can provide a range of choices so individual children can find challenges that match their interests and ability. These can include materials for "open-ended" activities (such as blocks and Play-Doh) that children can structure themselves, "problem-posing" tasks that can be solved in different ways (such as art activities and certain construction activities), and "closed-ended" activities (such as puzzles and matching games) that have clear goals and require several steps to reach them.

In addition to offering appropriate materials and opportunities for choice, adults can assist self-direction by providing sufficient time for children to carry out chosen activities and can protect them from unnecessary interference or distractions. It is frustrating for children when their ongoing activities are cut off before they are finished. Choice periods that are too brief cannot promote deepening concentration and task involvement.

Protecting children from unnecessary interference while they are involved in cognitive activities also encourages a longer focus on tasks and resistance to distraction. Adults can refrain from interrupting children and can discourage peers from doing so. Ground rules can stipulate that children need not relinquish materials to others before they have finished with them or reached their goal. Requiring a young child to "share" a puzzle when she is in the midst of trying to master it discourages focused involvement and goal orientation. Although it may be necessary to allot timed periods of access to popular activity centers, such as block and dramatic play areas, these should be long enough for children to experience the rewards of carrying out a process or goal-oriented activity.

Play areas or centers can also be designed to support and protect focused involvement. They can be arranged to accommodate the types of activities they contain (larger areas for blocks, for instance) and sheltered from neighboring spaces with shelves or walls. To prevent crowding, ground rules can stipulate the number of children allowed in an area at one time. Planning boards, which children use to specify the area where they will play, or similar self-monitoring techniques can allow children to control such numbers without adult assistance. Needed materials can also be available to children so they can carry out activities independently. They should not have to ask adults for materials needed to carry out the various activities in the environment. If collage making is an available choice, for instance, all materials needed for this activity (paper, paste, scissors, and other two- or three-dimensional materials for collages) should be within the children's reach. Independent access to these materials helps children to organize their own activities and develop the ability to plan ahead. They can think about the things they need to carry out an activity and can gather them together before beginning.

Assisting Learning

Caregivers also support self-regulation in cognitive activities by actively encouraging independence and persistence, by teaching techniques that give children strategies for problem solving, and by providing assistance in ways that preserve children's goals and feelings of control.

In addition to providing an environment that supports self-regulated action, adults can encourage independent effort and persistence. It is important to distinguish between appropriate attention and responsiveness to children from behaviors that encourage dependence. Children may ask for "help" from adults when they really want attention. Adults can respond by giving attention but not unneeded help. For instance, a child may ask a caregiver to help her "draw a picture" or "do the Lego." The adult can probe to see whether help is really needed by asking what the child is having trouble doing. If there is a genuine difficulty (the child may want to make a dog or a hat but not know how to begin, or may not be able to make the Lego pieces stick together), the adult can address the problem. The adult can model techniques or describe a strategy that enables the child to do the task. If the child does not really need help, the caregiver can try to clarify the actual request ("I don't think you need help with this—did you want company?"). He or she can respond to the child's request for attention or company by joining her or by explaining why it is not possible at this time. The adult can also suggest a peer as an alternative companion.

It is often difficult for caregivers to resist providing help as soon as they see a child struggling. However, working through difficulties to solve a problem or master a task independently increases children's persistence and feelings of competence. It is important that the challenge be appropriate for the child's level of skill so that she has a good chance of ultimate success.

If it becomes clear that a child does need help, caregivers can provide it in ways that preserve persistent effort and feelings of competence while offering the strategies needed for success. Observation of the child's efforts can usually reveal the source of the problem. Assistance can then be provided in the form of questions, suggested strategies, or modeled techniques. For instance, a child may be trying to match pictures and is becoming confused and trying some alternatives over and over. The adult can ask, "Which picture do you want to match first?" and then, when the child has selected one, can suggest, "Put each card that doesn't match over here (on the side) so you know which ones you've tried." If the child is still overwhelmed after attempting to use this approach, the adult can simplify the task by reducing the number of alternatives ("How about matching this group first? Then we can add the rest"). These approaches provide "scaffolds" for the child's efforts, but it is still the child and not the adult who is carrying out the activity. In addition, the adult has contributed to the child's ability to carry out the activity independently in the future by providing strategies she can implement herself.

When presenting unfamiliar materials or tasks to children, adults can include the strategies that will help them use the materials successfully and perform the tasks independently. In addition to modeled demonstrations, simple verbal descriptions of steps and strategies that children can later give themselves in "private speech" are increasingly helpful. When doing a puzzle, for instance, children can learn general puzzle strategies ("Lay all the pieces out so you can see them," "Try the edge pieces first," "Turn pieces around to see whether they fit another way," "Think of the picture this puzzle makes"), and as well as more task-specific strategies ("The wheels of the car fit on the bottom," "The parts of the dog go together").

When learning to play a group game, children need to understand the goal and the steps in the process. Descriptions of these can be more detailed for older children, but, in general, such descriptions help everyone to know what they are trying to do, how an activity is related to things they know how to do, and the strategies they need to do it. When teaching children to play Lotto, for instance, adults can explain the type of activity while showing the materials ("This is a matching game. There are big cards with many pictures and little cards with just one picture"). The goal and the steps to reach it can then be described ("In this game you put the little cards on the pictures of the big card that match. Everyone gets a big card. I will hold up the little cards one at a time, and you see whether you have the matching picture on your big card. If you do, you get the little card to put on the match. You are finished when all the pictures on your big card are covered with matching little cards"). Younger children may need to see each step carried out as it is described, while older children may soon be able to do the activity without adult help.

A number of tasks can be carried out in more than one way, and children can "construct" strategies and solutions to various problems. There is more than one way to draw a person or build a tower, and children's self-regulatory skills are improved by opportunities to experiment and invent. They can do this independently, in "cooperative learning" projects with other children, and in individual or group "problem-solving" sessions with adults. Adults can pose problems that are real in the environment ("The gerbil likes to be out of the cage, but he keeps running away. How could we build a play area for him that will keep him safe and stop him from running away?"). They can also pose interesting new problems ("It is a windy day. How could we make kites that will really fly?"). There is not one "right" solution to these problems, and children can experiment with different ideas. Adults can also use questioning techniques to assist children as they think about possible solutions or try out their ideas ("Do you think the gerbil could climb over that wall?" "Why/why not?" "How will you hold onto the kite you have made?"). Problem-posing and questioning techniques help children to become aware of the problem-solving process itself, and of their own (executive) decision-making processes (Casey & Tucker, 1994).

Motivation for Self-Regulation

Research suggests that certain caregiver behaviors, characteristics of the physical environment, and children's own perception of themselves influence motivation for self-regulation. Motivation for both self-control and mastery is affected by (1) family environments and child-rearing practices, (2) the range of options, challenges, expectations, and support systems in particular environments, and (3) a child's perception of her own competence and internal control (Harter, 1981, 1992; Skinner et al., 1998). Suggestions for supporting and increasing this motivation, in relation to these findings, are offered in the following paragraphs.

Child-Rearing Practices

A number of parental behaviors have been associated with motivation for control and mastery in children:

1. To develop and support motivation for self-regulation, caregivers can relate to children in *caring* and emotionally supportive ways.
2. They can interact with children in ways that are *responsive* to their activities and communications, showing children that their activities make an impact on the social environment and that their social communications are effective.
3. Caregivers can give *consistent*, but not rigid, responses to children's behavior that help them understand what behaviors, attitudes, and achievements are appropriate and valued.
4. They can use *inductive guidance strategies* that focus on connections between cause and effect and use problem-solving techniques to resolve disciplinary or social problems.
5. They can *encourage responsibility and independence* by providing appropriate opportunities to act in these ways and demonstrating support and approbation for children's efforts.
6. When children need assistance, caregivers can *teach problem-solving strategies* in ways that add to rather than decrease their independence.

The Environment (Coherence, Choice, Challenge, Expectations, Support)

A primary requirement for fostering motivation for self-regulation is providing an environment *coherent* enough that the standards for self-regulated action are clear and the outcomes of these actions can be reasonably predicted. In order to choose goals independently and work persistently toward reaching them, children have to understand the range of options available to them and the probable consequences of reaching the goals they choose. They need to know what activities they can appropriately engage in, which they are permitted to carry out independently of adults, what range of strategies they can use, and what kinds of outcomes are acceptable. Many of these change with age and experience, so some standards of behavior and achievement are constantly evolving.

Five-year-olds are given a broader range of *choices* and are permitted to carry out more of them independently than 3-year-olds. At the age of 5 a child may be allowed to wash dishes in the sink with adult help or to set the table by herself, whereas a 3-year-old may be permitted only to dry unbreakable dishes or may be given the napkins to put on the table. The range of choices a child can be appropriately given depend on her level of skill. If children are consistently allowed or encouraged to attempt tasks they cannot carry out successfully, their feelings of competence and efficacy will suffer and motivation to engage in these tasks will be reduced.

It is not necessary to succeed every time. Tasks that are too easy (require too little effort) do not encourage motivation for self-regulation (Dweck & Elliott, 1983). They do not present an appropriate level of *challenge* and may not be interesting. The most motivating tasks are those that are difficult enough to present a challenge but promise a good chance of success (Redding et al., 1988). Children who do not feel competent are more likely to choose tasks that are below their actual level of skill.

Children also need to understand adult restrictions and *expectations* about task performance. They must know what strategies they are allowed to use to carry out tasks. Stepping on a puzzle piece to force it into place is typically not permitted, for instance, whereas turning it around to see whether it fits at a different angle is encouraged. Children are often motivated to engage in experiments with materials that are not appropriate to the setting or to the material. They may want to build a tall block tower and then knock it over, which is not safe in settings where people or other objects might be injured. They may be interested in using small metal cars in sand or water, which could damage them, or painting over posters on the wall. In many cases children use materials inappropriately through ignorance of possible negative outcomes. They may not realize that glue will be hard to get off a computer or that paint can stain a rug.

Negative outcomes and restrictions with a negative tone—that focus on prohibitions rather than opportunities—can reduce motivation to engage in self-directed activities or may create rebellion. Alternative approaches that *support* motivation are similar to those that help children control behavior and emotional responses:

1. Adults can prepare the environment (especially the play environment) so that it includes a variety of activities children can safely and productively carry out, and excludes opportunities

for activities that are prohibited and materials children are not supposed to touch.

2. A small set of reasonable (for both adults and children) ground rules can minimize the need for adult intervention and restriction and maximize children's sense of control and mastery. When these guidelines focus on what children are *permitted* to do rather than on what is forbidden (e.g., "We walk inside" rather than "No running") there is a more positive "climate" for action.

3. Self-confidence and self-direction are also bolstered when adults respect children's ideas for activities, even when they are problematic, and use problem solving to find alternate ways of carrying them out. It *is permissible* for block towers to be knocked down outdoors, for instance, if other children stay clear of the action when this is done. When children find that their plans of action can work when they are carefully thought out, they are more likely to do such planning themselves in the future.

Enhancing Perception of Competence and Control

Motivation for self-regulation is positively related to children's perception of their own competence and ability to exercise control. They develop such perceptions in interaction with other people, objects, and mastery opportunities in the environment. When caregivers' responses are caring, contingent (on child activities), and appropriate, children develop a sense of agency and control (Skinner et al., 1998). Children also develop a sense of agency when they are able to manipulate and master objects or tasks. They feel competent when they are successful in their interactions with the social and physical environment. If they are more successful in one of these areas, they will feel more competent in that area.

When caregivers allow and expect children to carry out age-appropriate activities independently, children develop similar expectations. If others help children with tasks they could do themselves, or do the tasks for them, children may feel that they are not capable of doing them. It may take longer for children to put on their own clothes, put away their toys, or help with a few household (or classroom) chores, but performing these activities helps them feel competent.

When children are having difficulties, the types of assistance strategies caregivers use influence perceived competence and control. If adults take over a task or give directions that require only compliance, children's perceived control is undermined. To support feelings of control while providing help, adults can use several strategies. They can ask questions, to help children discover their own solutions to problems, or provide strategies that children can implement independently. For instance, if a child asks for help because a block tower keeps falling down, the adult might ask, "How did you build it when it stayed up longest (or when you built the highest tower)?" or can suggest, "It usually helps to put the bigger blocks on the bottom." These approaches help the child begin to analyze the requirements of the task and provide strategies to use in the future.

Other people's responses to children's efforts and achievements are also important. If the standards and expectations of significant others, especially caregivers, exceed a child's ability, she will not feel competent even if she performs at an age-appropriate level. If, for instance, a child prints the first letter of her name after great effort and a parent asks, "Where's the rest?" the child will not feel competent. High expectations support motivation when the level of challenge requires effort but is within the child's capacity.

Evaluative comments set or influence the standards the child will try to meet. Those that focus attention on pleasing the adult ("I really like the way you built that tower," "I like Janie's picture best") suggest that this is the primary goal of the task. Those that focus on competition ("Tanya finished the most puzzles," "Jaimie's story is the longest," "José remembered more zoo animals than anyone else") establish outdoing others as a primary goal. Because not all can be "first" or please the adult equally, perceived competence will be diminished for many.

Vague or general evaluations ("That's great," "You did that wrong") do not provide much information to the child about her competence. Adult comments are more effective in supporting self-regulation when they focus on specific aspects of what the child has done. General comments such as "Good job" tell the child nothing about what parts of the "job" were "good." Specific comments can recognize the child's effort ("You really worked hard on that painting"), persistence ("That puzzle was hard and it took a long time, but you kept going till you finished it") or achievement ("You matched every pair correctly," "You mixed blue and yellow and made green," "You wrote all the letters of your name"). Such comments can help the child notice progress ("You remembered two new colors today—purple and orange," "Now you know the letters of your last name too") or aspects of her task that might be improved ("If you put in the last three pieces, the puzzle will be finished," "Most of the blocks are picked up, but two are still under the shelf"). By noticing specific features, the adult brings them to the child's attention and consciousness and provides evaluative information or feedback that can be useful for self-regulation in the future.

Table 8.1 summarizes the types of self-regulation that are developing during the preschool and kindergarten years and the major environmental influences that contribute to development.

SUMMARY

Preschool and kindergarten children are increasingly capable of voluntary internal self-regulation in both social and cognitive areas. In a widening range of situations and with increasing reliability they can manage their emotional responses, comply with age-appropriate rules and directions, and independently carry out problem solving and mastery tasks. In addition, they are interested in other children and are developing self-regulated strategies for successful and cooperative social interaction. They are internalizing social rules and attitudes and developing consistent styles of interaction, including prosocial or antisocial dispositions. Motivation for self-regulation also increases during this period if children feel competent and able to direct themselves.

The environment supports the continuing growth of emotional, behavioral, prosocial, and cognitive control. It also influences motivation for control. The emotional climate of the family and the guidance strategies, expectations, and teaching strategies of parents and other adults continue of be of central importance. In addition, peer and media influences have an increasing impact as children's experiences expand. Aspects of the physical environment can also help or hinder children's attempts to explore and master it.

A warm and responsive social climate in group care and education settings, as well as within the family, continues to support the

TABLE 8.1. Developmental Milestones of Self-Regulation in Preschool and Kindergarten Children and Major Environmental Supports

Domain of development	Milestones	Role of adults	Role of environment
Social/ emotional behavior	More capable of controlling emotions, abiding by rules, and refraining from forbidden behaviors More capable of using language to regulate own behavior and influence others More interest in peers and peer acceptance, so more apt to regulate self in relation to peers More capable of cooperative interaction with peers Can learn more effective interaction strategies Can engage in dramatic play with roles and rules	Function as models, resources, and guides for: • social interaction styles and strategies • self-control strategies • values and attitudes Use responsive guidance techniques that: • use language to assist self-control • emphasize individual control over behavior • support developing inner controls • give reasons for desired behaviors • suggest appropriate strategies in context Supervise play with peers and help to resolve or negotiate conflicts when necessary (using a problem-solving approach) Provide opportunities for dramatic play and for choice among appropriate alternatives	Contains a trusted adult to support independence, self-control, and appropriate interactions with peers Contains clear guidelines (appropriate for age and developmental level of the child or children) for responsibilities, opportunities (choices), expectations, and consequences that are consistently and appropriately implemented Provides opportunities for supervised interactions with peers Contains materials that support constructive peer interaction and dramatic play Minimizes exposure to negative behaviors and attitudes
Prosocial behavior	Begins to talk about mental states of self and others Better understanding of how others may feel Can engage in deliberate helping, sharing, and comforting behaviors Internalizing standards of behavior Developing more stable prosocial (or antisocial) attitudes and behaviors	Model prosocial attitudes and behaviors Minimize exposure to violent or antisocial models (live or media) Attribute prosocial motives to children Assign appropriate responsibilities to children Expect and encourage responsible behavior Provide guidelines for behavior that connect behavior with its effects and include the consequences of behaviors for others	Provides opportunities for positive and cooperative interactions with others Includes materials and activities that encourage and support cooperative and prosocial behaviors and attitudes Provides guidelines that require, encourage, and support responsibility, respect, and care for others, and positive interaction styles Sanctions negative or antisocial behavior

TABLE 8.1 (*continued*)

Domain of development	Milestones	Role of adults	Role of environment
Cognitive self-regulation	Can engage in a wider range of cognitive activities More able to carry out multistep activities More able to control attention and resist distraction Can learn to use more advanced task attack and problem-solving strategies More able to choose tasks appropriate for own level of skill (from among familiar alternatives)	Provide developmentally appropriate play materials and activities that support: • appropriate choice • developing learning and problem-solving strategies • engaging in multistep activities • attention focus and control • construction of cognitive categories that mediate understanding of order, structure, predictability in the environment Model and communicate effective language Use "scaffolding" to broaden children's understanding and provide assistance (including suggesting appropriate task attack and problem-solving strategies in context)	Coherent and predictable enough for the child to comprehend the order and predictability Flexible enough for the child to appropriately influence or affect aspects of the environment Contains an appropriate range of materials for child's interests and abilities Provides for choice within interest and ability range Provides time for choice and carrying out chosen activities Contains space and opportunity for action and investigation, with protected spaces for uninterrupted, focused activities
Motivation for self-regulation	Moving from a primary focus on exploration in tasks to a focus on mastery and reaching chosen goals Moving from primary interest in process of doing tasks to products produced Beginning to evaluate own competence in relation to: • reaching chosen goals • evaluations of other • success of others	Demonstrate reinforcing attitudes toward independence, persistence, and mastery efforts Design the environment for independence Design materials and activities so that a child or small group can carry them out without constant direction from others Protect the child's focused involvement and independent action Use assistance strategies that protect the child's independent focus and agency (including providing strategies the child can later use independently)	Contains enough coherence, predictability, and flexibility that the child can both understand what is expected and engage in independent self-regulated action Provides appropriate level of challenges to match the child's interests and abilities Provides materials that the child can structure independently Contains opportunities to practice self-regulation and choice Provides materials that the child can access and use independently In group settings, provides rules that support and protect independent action (such as provision for independent or small-group focused activities and guidelines on how many can occupy an interest area) Includes techniques for independent organization of activities (such as planning or choice boards)

development of self-regulation in all areas. Adult models help children learn both how to behave and how to think. During the preschool and kindergarten years children are internalizing their understanding of the behavior and attitudes (values and beliefs) of the important people in their lives.

Self-regulation is further supported when caregivers encourage independence and give children responsibility for age- and skill-appropriate tasks. Attributing positive skills, attitudes, and motives to children is also helpful. When these attributions are accompanied by a reasonable amount of success in the children's own experience, they come to expect themselves to be capable, responsible, and motivated to carry out self-regulated and responsible actions. They are also more likely to actually perform such actions.

Guidance strategies that help children understand cause–effect relationships and provide reasons for rules help children to learn to guide themselves. Teaching and assistance strategies that help children feel competent and help them engage in independent social, mastery, and problem solving activities also help to increase self-regulation and self-confidence.

Environments that nurture self-regulation are orderly and consistent enough for children to understand the requirements for successful independent functioning within them. They provide appropriate ground rules for action that allow children to carry out a variety of activities, alone or with peers, without the need for constant adult control. The materials and activities in these environments are also designed to interest and challenge children and to support self-regulated activities.

9

Supporting Self-Regulation
in Primary School Children

OVERVIEW OF DEVELOPMENTAL
AND ENVIRONMENTAL INFLUENCES

Most executive self-regulatory functions are well under way by the
primary school years, although they may not be fully internalized until early adolescence (Barkley, 1997). Between the fifth and seventh
year of age, there is a noticeable increase in self-regulation (Berkowitz, 1982) and shifts in mental functioning have been noted by a
number of psychologists with a developmental focus (Erikson, 1963;
Freud, 1920; Piaget, 1970; White, 1970). During this period children
become more responsible and more consciously aware of their actions and thoughts. Self-speech becomes internalized between the
ages of 6 and 9 (Berk, 1992). Over these years the development of
self-regulation continues to be assisted by a warm and supportive social climate, a coherent physical environment that is challenging and
supportive of independent action, and adults who encourage responsibility and independence and teach effective control strategies. In addition, the development of self-regulation can now be assisted by
nurturing children's conscious awareness and conscious use of their

own executive skills and processes (Donaldson, 1978; Zimmerman et al., 1996).

The environment has a major impact on the self-regulatory skills children bring to school and continues to influence their development in the primary years. Although the family continues to be important, school and peer experiences become very powerful during this period. As children's activities expand into a widening world, a larger group of people and events help to shape their development. Children are also increasingly aware of and interested in these outside influences. They seek feedback on their actions and products from the people and achievement criteria available in their expanding world and increasingly judge themselves according to standards based on this information.

Cognitive Development

Cognitive self-regulation is of growing importance during the elementary school years and is increasingly emphasized in school reform proposals. Research over the last 15 years has suggested that a major source of the differences between high- and low-achieving students is the degree to which they become regulators of their own learning (Meichenbaum, 1984; Pressley et al., 1990; Zimmerman & Schunk, 1989).

The environment has a major effect on the development of cognitive self-regulation, especially conscious (metacognitive) control of thinking and learning. Language appears to support this development (Berk, 1992; Berk & Winsler, 1995; Rogoff, 1990), as Vygotsky (1962) suggested, but literacy (Donaldson, 1978) and Western-style schooling also appear to play important roles (Cole, 1992; Cole et al., 1971; Cole & Scribner, 1974; Farnham-Diggory, 1992; Sternberg, 1987). Children can be taught strategies that they can consciously and voluntarily use to assist control of behavior and cognitive processes such as memory and problem solving. A variety of programs for teaching these strategies have been suggested (Baldwin & Baldwin, 1998; Barkley, 1998; Hughes, 1988; Logue, 1995; Zimmerman et al., 1996). The programs provide different rationales about why they are effective, based on behavioral, social learning, or Vygotskian theory, but their training approaches are similar. Verbal strategies for self-instruction are taught, and the child is expected to use them in private speech to guide behavior. Literacy may also assist metacognitive awareness by separating thinking from immediate experience and facilitating conscious reflection upon, and comparison among, a variety of concepts and alternatives (Donaldson, 1978).

Children's growing awareness of themselves makes them particularly vulnerable to challenges and judgments in the environment. Their perceived successes and failures and the perceived judgments of others are internalized and affect motivation. When children believe that they are competent and able to control important aspects of their lives, motivation to exercise this control increases (Deci & Ryan, 1985, 1987). When they believe that they are able to control the outcome of school tasks, they are more interested in these activities and more persistent in pursuing them (Dweck, 1991; Harter, 1981, 1992). When they believe in their competence and control in any area of functioning, they are more motivated to engage in it (Skinner, 1986; Skinner et al., 1998). Interactions with adults and peers and children's own performance in tasks (including school tasks, sports activities, and artistic or other creative efforts) affect their perceived control and sense of competence. Lack of success in their efforts or negative external judgments can reduce children's positive beliefs about themselves. Even children who are objectively competent in school do less well when they doubt their abilities (Miserandino, 1996). Children in this age range are just developing internal standards for achievement, so they are particularly vulnerable to external expectations and evaluations.

Social Development

Emotional control and the ability to conform to external rules of behavior are required of children as they reach school age. In the primary school setting they are expected to be able to control emotional outbursts and aggression, conform to school rules, and interact cooperatively with other children (Bowman & Svetina, 1992). Teachers value positive and cooperative behavior, regulation of emotions, and the ability to follow classroom rules and adult requests (Alexander & Entwisle, 1988; McKim & Cowen, 1987; Pallas et al., 1987; Reynolds, 1991). Failure in these social–emotional areas, as well as in cognitive areas, results in negative teacher evaluations and placement in special classrooms (Fry, 1984). Teachers' ratings of "conduct" during the primary school years are predictive of later academic performance (Entwisle & Hayduk, 1982).

If not corrected, early social problems, such as lack of appropriate behavior and emotional control or lack of positive skills for approaching and interacting with peers, tend to follow children into elementary school and beyond (Coie & Dodge, 1983; Parker & Asher, 1987; Putallaz & Gottman, 1981). The ability to form positive and appropriate relationships with peers is as important as the ability to comply with school rules and interact positively with adults. Peer acceptance is extremely important to children from primary school onward, and peer rejection is associated with a variety of negative outcomes in school and in later life (Achenbach & Edelbrock, 1981, 1991). Prosocial behavior and social competence, which includes positive and effective strategies for interacting with others, are related to each other and to peer acceptance (Dodge et al., 1986; Howes, 1990; Katz & McClellan, 1997). Lack of social competence and frequent aggression are related to peer rejection, and to a number of associated psychological problems, in both early and later years (Achenback & Edelbrock, 1981, 1991).

Early social experiences affect children's expectations and behavior in primary school. These experiences are transformed into internalized models for self-guidance, or "generalized cognitive representations of relationships" (Rudolph et al., 1995), which affect the way they behave and interpret the behaviors of others. Continuing experiences can influence these models, but established tendencies are increasingly hard to change. Children's ongoing self-directed behavior is guided by their expectations about the social and physical environment and about their own capabilities in it, and their interpretations of other peoples' behavior is filtered through these perceptions, so previous patterns of action and reaction tend to recur.

During the early elementary years children become more consciously aware of themselves and of their relationships with others. They are more vulnerable to external judgments and increasingly susceptible to the judgments of peers. As children become more involved in peer-regulated activities, they are increasingly influenced by the norms of the group. It is harder for them to resist behaviors that "everybody else" is doing and attitudes that peers do not share. They do not want to be "left out" or thought to be too different. As peer influences become stronger, children who have learned to be responsible and independent, and who have close, positive relationships with families that provide firm but not oppressive guidance, are less vulnerable to negative peer influences (Kandel & Lesser, 1972).

Media and other influences outside the family also become more important to children, as well as increasingly accessible to them. Children of this age are exposed to a larger number and variety of models of behavior and thinking, which provide both opportunity and risk. As children become more independent, families are not always aware of the range of influences that may affect them. Open lines of communication and frequent discussions with trusted adults help maintain support for the types of self-regulation parents and teachers want to foster.

School-age children are considered accountable for their actions in ways that younger children are not. They are expected to know right from wrong in the circumstances of their daily lives, and their understanding is expected to have a moral dimension. They are considered to have a conscience and to feel guilt when they violate standards. Children in this age range are very interested in fairness and reciprocity, but their judgments are still relatively primitive (Hoffman, 1983, 1987; Kohlberg, 1969; Piaget, 1965). Their understanding of the (moral) principles on which a number of social decisions are based reflects their (still immature) level of cognitive development and relative lack of experience. Children are now capable of making and sticking to rules, but may apply them in ways that are rigid or even punitive. Previously learned prosocial or antisocial dispositions also affect their judgments. Children can benefit from discussions with peers to help them understand differing perspectives (Piaget, 1965, 1967). In addition, adults can help to scaffold increased understanding by participating in problem-solving discussions with children (Berk & Winsler, 1995; Katz & McClellan, 1997).

School Reform

As the body of information to be acquired by students increases geometrically, and as real-life work skills increasingly require the ability to learn new skills and adapt to new situations, there is a growing dissatisfaction with a transfer-of-facts approach to teaching and learning. School systems are searching for ways to promote the types of skills that will support a lifetime of self-initiated, self-regulated learning (Biemiller & Meichenbaum, 1992; Zimmerman & Schunk, 1989). They are realizing that children must be able to generalize beyond content that may become obsolete and to develop skills that enable them to become lifelong learners.

Many who are interested in reform have suggested that effective educational practice throughout formal schooling should focus on developing self-regulated learning skills such as goal setting, problem solving, planning, collaborating, and self-evaluation (American Psychological Association, 1993; Graham et al., 1992; Zimmerman & Schunk, 1989). A number of psychologists with differing theoretical perspectives are focusing on the importance of self-regulation and how it can be achieved (Barkley, 1997; Logue, 1995; Zimmerman et al., 1996).

Unlike previous models of school reform, an emphasis on self-regulation focuses on *how* students achieve, in both social and solitary settings, and view learning as something that happens *by* rather than *to* them (Zimmerman, 1986, 1989). Research indicates that most teachers want children to become participants in their own learning—to be willing and able to take responsibility for regulating their own academic achievements (Corno, 1992). They believe that children's ability to monitor and regulate their own learning is at least as important to achievement as their cognitive abilities (Pintrich & Degroot, 1990; Schunk & Zimmerman, 1994). Psychologists have described self-regulated learners as "metacognitively, motivationally, and behaviorally active participants in their own learning" (Zimmerman, 1989, p. 4), who "know how to plan, allocate resources, seek help, and correct their own work" (Paris & Ayres, 1994, p. 28).

Motivation is an important component of most formulations. A number of psychologists have emphasized the value of intrinsic motivation because it results in a preference for tasks with choice, challenge, and control (Stipek, 1993). They have stressed the importance of purpose, direction, and force in students' efforts (Paris & Ayres, 1994). As children mature, the need to feel competent differentiates into motivation for competence and achievement in specific areas (Deci & Porak, 1978). During the early elementary years children are also developing standards for judging the adequacy of their achievements (Zimmerman & Schunk, 1989; Zimmerman et al., 1996). Children who believe that they are academically competent are more interested in school learning activities (Harter, 1981, 1992). Experiences of being successful in mastering challenges and meeting internal standards increase the feeling of competence and the motivation to engage in these activities. Experiences of failure decrease feelings of competence and motivation to try.

APPLICATIONS TO PRACTICE

Primary school children's expanding social and cognitive world presents both increased opportunities and increased risks for their developing self-regulatory control. Children in this age range are given a wider variety of opportunities to exercise and learn self-regulation, but the environment also presents a growing number of influences and challenges that can undermine real and perceived control. The following sections discuss both opportunities and risks in the four areas of self-regulatory development that have been the focus of previous chapters: (1) social and emotional behavior, (2) prosocial dispositions and behavior, (3) cognitive self-regulation, and (4) motivation for self-regulation.

Social and Emotional Behavior

Primary school children are better able to regulate their emotions and behaviors than younger children, partially because they have greater cognitive capacities. They understand that emotions have to be regulated. They are also more able to interpret what is causing arousal and what needs to be done about it, and are better able to do what is required (Garber et al., 1991). They have developed more internal "problem-focused," rather than external "emotion focused," strategies to regulate emotions (Brenner & Salovey, 1993) and are capable of conscious self-control (Mischel & Mischel, 1977). They can reflect and make deliberate decisions about what they should do in particular situations. This allows them to learn from discussions with others as well as from concrete experiences and to profit from everyday experiences in more complex ways.

Primary school children can reflect on their own and others' behaviors and the consequences of these behaviors in the environment. They can also evaluate these behaviors and consequences against developing internal standards for performance (Bandura, 1997). They are beginning to understand the perspectives of others and are capable of rule-governed behavior (Piaget, 1965; Piaget & Inhelder, 1969). These cognitive abilities support more sophisticated internal techniques for controlling behavior and emotions. They also allow adults to use guidance strategies that assume interest in general principles and rely more on children's ability to understand the reasons for their own and other's behaviors. Problem-solving discussions can now go beyond specific instances of behavior and specific problems to more general issues, standards, and rules. They can include references to internal standards ("What do you think you should do/ should be done in situations like this?" "What do you think about the decision you made?") and hypothetical possibilities ("Is there another way you could have dealt with that?" "Do you think things would be different if she had apologized?" "What do you think should be done if someone wants to join the game but doesn't know how to play very well?"). Primary school children are also better able to resolve disputes with peers without (or with less) adult intervention or facilitation and can learn more from these negotiations. Parents and teachers can reduce the power of negative peer or media examples by discussion and example, especially if children have learned to trust and respect them in earlier years.

Adults can also assist the development of self-regulated social skills by structuring the environment to allow and support positive activities with others. They can arrange schedules that include adequate time for self-directed social experiences and provide materials and situations that support such experiences. Social interest is high during these years, and social skills are critical for positive school and life outcomes. The classroom environment should include an emphasis on developing social as well as cognitive skills, especially because they are interrelated throughout early childhood (Berk & Winsler, 1995; Katz & McClellan, 1997).

Classroom schedules can include both unstructured free time for voluntary social activities and more structured cooperative learning periods. Many social activities preferred by this age group, such as board games and joint computer activities, can also be cognitive learning activities (Bronson, 1995). Teachers can select games and computer activities for free choice periods that support educational as well as social goals. Children may "enjoy" activities that are unproductive or lead to negative outcomes (such as violent video games), so interest alone is not a sufficient criterion. An overemphasis on competition can also be counterproductive at these ages, because children's understanding of rules can be overcome by their desire to win. They may resort to cheating when the emphasized goal is being "first."

Cooperative learning activities support both social and cognitive development (Johnson, 1991; Johnson, Johnson, Johnson-Holubee, & Roy, 1984). They emphasize discussion and joint problem solving, which can help bring social, problem-solving and decision-making processes to conscious awareness. Even when children work individually on projects or tasks, their awareness and conscious understanding of what they have done can be enhanced when they share their experiences with others in follow-up discussions.

Generally, parents and teachers can provide a climate of respect, acceptance, and positive expectations for self-regulated behavior. They can model positive and appropriate behaviors and attitudes and use guidance strategies that support social problem solving and understanding. They can allow children to attempt to solve their own problems whenever possible, suggesting or modeling problem-solving and negotiation strategies, or use strategies that promote cooperative interaction in situations where adult intervention can support growth. During the early elementary years (and beyond), parents and teachers can also be alert for opportunities to bring children's interaction strategies and decision-making processes to consciousness, so that children can learn to control and direct them more effectively.

Prosocial Dispositions and Behavior

The family climate and guidance strategies used by parents continue to be important for supporting prosocial dispositions in primary school children. However, school and peer experiences are now central in their lives and exert a powerful influence on them. Children who have internalized prosocial attitudes and values from their families are more resistant to negative external influences, especially if warm, responsive, and trusting relationships with parents continue and parents keep expecting and encouraging responsible and prosocial behavior.

Parents can continue to monitor influences and events in children's larger environments, helping them to interpret challenges to the prosocial values and behaviors parents wish to support and guiding them (when possible) away from experiences they believe will be harmful. Some peer or media experiences that may be appropriate for older children—and might even challenge older children to reach higher levels of social understanding—can confuse or frighten younger, less mature and experienced children. It is very difficult for parents to resist what they believe to be inappropriate or negative influences in the peer or media environment. It requires tact, respect, trust, open lines of communication between parents and children, and adult understanding of the importance of these experiences to children.

Children are increasingly drawn to peers as they move toward greater independence from the family, and their perception of their own competence is related to their relationships with peers. Relationships with peers are a source of support and reassurance as they move into a larger and less familiar world. Doing what others do and "fitting in" may appear to be a safely net as well as a challenge. Resisting peer or other social influences that challenge previously internalized attitudes and beliefs, requires confidence in one's own self-regulatory abilities. Children who feel competent and in control are less likely to behave in ways they believe are inappropriate or wrong.

Certain types of school programs and teaching techniques also appear to support prosocial dispositions and behaviors. Cooperative learning techniques that reduce the negative aspects of competition and promote cooperation reduce conflict and increase prosocial behaviors such as helping (Hertz-Lazarowitz & Sharan, 1984). When school programs include cooperative activities, efforts to promote social understanding, modeled prosocial behaviors, encouragement to engage in these behaviors, and discipline techniques that emphasize self-control, "moral" principles, and student participation in decision making (empowerment and control), prosocial behaviors increase (Solomon et al., 1990). These techniques are very similar to the guidance strategies for parents suggested by the Zahn-Waxler/Radke-Yarrow research (1979, 1992) to promote prosocial behavior in children.

One comprehensive school in California implemented a program that included these components in a longitudinal intervention with children of kindergarten age through third grade (see the program description in Chapter 4, pp. 106–107). Children in this program, in comparison to children in several similar schools without this program, showed an increase in prosocial behaviors, the use of social problem-solving strategies, planning, compromise, and concern for the needs of others. The program emphasized the development of inner control, personal responsibility, and intrinsic motivation for academic achievement as well as prosocial behavior. It used techniques such as group discussions, modeling, and adult encouragement. The emphasis on developing inner control and intrinsic motivation contrasts with programs suggested by behavioral theorists that are designed to "reduce impulsivity" and teach children to wait for delayed rewards (Logue, 1995). It assumes that the primary school child is capable of altruism (caring for others), moral understanding of reciprocity, intrinsic interest in doing well (for oneself) and doing good (to others), and cognitive control over behavior.

Cognitive Self-Regulation

Maturing executive functions in the brain support the marked increase in capacity for self-regulation that occurs in the early primary school years. Children can now mentally represent information in ways that allow planning for more delayed goals and decrease the need for immediate rewards. Their private speech is also less designed to control immediate behavior than to invoke and use more general strategies of problem solving such as self-questioning, problem clarification, and reflecting on possible rules (Barkley, 1997).

Primary school children's cognitive abilities include a growing (metacognitive) awareness of their own thinking processes and the possibility of controlling them. They are conscious of their self-speech and can learn ways of using it to support control (Flavell et al., 1997). They are also beginning to think silently in words. Children can now learn strategies for *conscious* voluntary control of thinking and learning. They can learn to consciously set goals, select appropriate strategies to reach the goals, monitor progress and revise their strategies when necessary, and control attention and motivation until a goal is reached. They are much better able to resist distraction than younger children.

Strategies that increase self-regulation in problem solving and learning have been called "self-instruction strategies" by behavioral psychologists (Meichenbaum, 1977, 1984; Meichenbaum & Asarow,

1979), "self-regulatory processes" or "skills" by social learning theorists (Zimmerman et al., 1996), and "self-guiding speech" by Vygotskians (Berk & Winsler, 1995). The behavioral approach is the most prescriptive and directive. Strategy statements modeled by teachers or trainers are learned by children as step-by-step guides to approaching tasks. These include *problem definition* statements ("What is my goal?" "What do I have to do?"), *planning and response guidance* statements ("What materials do I need to do this?" "What should I do first?" "I need to work carefully"), *self-reinforcement* statements ("I know how to do this"), *self-evaluative* statements ("Am I doing this in the right order?" "Have I finished all the parts?"), and *coping* statements ("I have to try again," "I need to get help") (Meichenbaum, 1984). It is assumed that this "verbal behavior" on the part of the child can be learned like any other response.

Teaching strategies based on Bandura's (1986) social learning theory focus on the processes children must engage in to regulate their own problem solving and learning (Zimmerman et al., 1996). These processes include many of the same functions included in Meichenbaum's (1984) behavioral model. *Goal setting, strategic planning, strategy implementation,* and *monitoring* (similar to *response guidance* in the behavioral model) are all addressed but the emphasis is on internal cognitive processes rather than learned instructions that direct task performance. The goal is to have the child, rather than the teacher, assume responsibility for and control of the learning process. Motivation and reward are conceived in terms of *self-efficacy perceptions* rather than *self-reinforcement.* Children learn to regulate their cognitive activities independently in order to reach self-selected goals (within curriculum guidelines) and internal performance standards. When they are successful in doing this, they are rewarded by feeling competent and effective.

Both behavioral and social learning theory approaches to teaching self-regulatory strategies assume that, as Vygotsky (1962) proposed, speech can be used by individuals to guide their own behavior. The Vygotskian approach focuses on the development of self-guiding private speech, which becomes "internalized" during the primary school years (Berk, 1992). The capacity for thinking in words gives children a powerful new tool. It assists memory and the representation of alternatives, making it possible to plan ahead and choose among alternative strategies or courses of action. It may also be a major mediator of "consciousness," because words make it easier for children to reflect on the contents of their minds. From the Vygotskian perspective, cognitive skills and self-regulatory strategies grow out of joint problem-solving experiences with adults or more experienced peers. Children internalize their own version (construction) of the strategies used by others, constantly improving them in further mentored experiences. They develop increasing control of thinking and learning processes as their strategies become increasingly adequate for independent functioning. The executive functions included in behavioral and social learning training programs are also considered important by Vygotskians, but their focus is on the social context of learning. There is an emphasis on "talk," on interactive experiences with others, and on "joint construction" (with others) of effective strategies for approaching tasks and problems. The goal is independent self-regulation, but the primary teaching strategy is collaboration.

The "reciprocal teaching" method suggested by Palincsar and Brown (1984) illustrates this approach. Although designed to promote comprehension of expository text in older (seventh-grade) children, the general method could be used with young children. The instructional strategy uses structured dialogues between teacher and child in which the teacher models comprehension questions about a story (essentially "who," "what," "when," and "why" questions) that scaffold the child's ability to reflect on the story herself and later use similar questions in private speech. In the Palincsar and Brown protocol the child and adult take turns "being the teacher" and asking comprehension questions, so the child co-constructs the comprehension process with the assistance of the adult.

From the Vygotskian perspective, all effective teaching supports the development of self-regulation because it is designed to increase a child's ability to carry out activities independently. Teachers, parents, or more experienced peers provide assistance at the point of difficulty for the child, in the context of real tasks and problems. Support is therefore provided in a child's "zone of proximal development" (in which she cannot move ahead independently but can with help). Optimally, the "help" is designed to give the child strategies that enable her to carry out the activity independently next time. This approach can provide targeted support for self-regulatory development in tasks because it focuses on providing appropriate strategies at the point where they are most needed, for an individual child in a particular situation. Strategies provided in the context of real problems are also more likely to be remembered and used in the future by children than those taught in the abstract, without a specific task- or problem-centered focus. They also preserve children's feelings of control and motivate them to "construct" an understanding of the concepts involved (Pressley et al., 1990; Pressley et al., 1992).

There is evidence to support the effectiveness of each of the three teaching approaches. In practice, behavioral training strategies are more often used for children with special needs or impulse control problems, and Vygotskian techniques are more often used in early childhood classrooms. It is possible that more cognitive maturity is required for the social learning theory approach than for behavioral or Vygotskian methods, as there is a greater emphasis on cognitive reflection and internalized standards of performance. Vygotskian scaffolding techniques can be used for children at any age, but with the emphasis on individualized support tailored to meet a child in her "zone of proximal development," they are more challenging to implement.

The classroom climate, rules, and opportunities also make a difference. For primary school children, as for younger children, opportunities for choice, experimentation, and independent problem solving support and promote the development of self-regulatory skills. A regimented classroom climate, in which all children are required to do the same thing at the same time in the same way, reduces feelings of control and discourages self-regulation. Providing a range of appropriate choices that allow children to reach curriculum goals in ways that are interesting to them and present challenges in an appropriate range of difficulty for their individual levels of skill, encourages goal setting, planning, monitoring, and persistence. When children feel self-directed they are more interested in reaching the goals they have chosen, invest more energy in pursuing them, and feel more responsible for the outcome.

Supporting Motivation for Self-Regulation

Strategies for control should be taught in ways that support the child's perception of competence and control. As children mature, the generalized need to feel competent differentiates into motivation for competence and achievement in specific areas (Deci & Porak, 1978). The primary school years are a period of particular vulnerability as children become more aware of themselves, of external standards, and of differences between themselves and others. They are increasingly motivated to engage in activities that they believe they do well and decreasingly motivated to do things they think they cannot do or cannot do adequately—in relation to others and to the standards of performance being internalized.

Children who believe they are academically competent are more interested in school learning activities (Harter, 1981, 1992). A sense of personal control also supports motivation (Deci & Ryan, 1985, 1987), and self-regulated learning gives students a sense of personal control (Zimmerman, 1985, 1995). Using external methods of control and providing rewards and punishments that enforce external control, such as threats and arbitrary deadlines (including speed tests and schedules for completion of tasks that have no relation to the tasks themselves or to individual differences), have detrimental effects on intrinsic motivation to learn and on self-directed learning (Lepper, 1981). The types of surveillance that imply external control are also detrimental (Deci & Ryan, 1987). Perceived external control diminishes feelings of personal responsibility for the outcomes of learning tasks and may make children feel helpless. When they do not feel able to control or influence the events that affect them, children are more likely to attribute their success to external factors like luck or teacher preference, and their failures to internal factors such as lack of ability (Dweck & Elliott, 1993). Children who feel helpless or incompetent avoid challenges and are less persistent.

Teachers can promote mastery-oriented motivation and self-regulated learning in the ways they assign tasks or goals, evaluate students, and provide help. They can provide tasks that are meaningful to children and explain the purposes and real-world significance of tasks when these are not obvious (Stipek, 1998). They can encourage personal goal setting and allow children to choose among an appropriate range of goals and tasks whenever possible. This approach can foster a sense of control and personal investment in the task or goal, as well as allow latitude for individual differences in interest and skill. Teachers can also allow children to use a range of different types of learning activities, producing a variety of products, to work toward specified classroom goals. The pace and time devoted to an activity or product can also vary, depending on a particular child's interest and skill. This provides opportunities for choice and self-direction and allows children with different interests and learning styles to do their best work. It can also minimize invidious comparisons.

The evaluation techniques used by teachers (or parents) have important effects on children's perception of their competence and control and, therefore, on their mastery motivation. Techniques that rely on individualized learning outcomes rather than comparative performance outcomes are more likely to support a child's intrinsic motivation in the task at hand and her motivation for self-regulated performance. Evaluation strategies that compare children in ways that produce winners and losers may make children feel inadequate and helpless. Their sense of control and interest in achievement is undermined when they are assigned an arbitrary rank or grade that places them on a continuum they may not understand and may feel they can do nothing to change. Under these circumstances rewards and punishments may appear arbitrary, determined by luck or chance, and external.

Stipek (1998) recommends a "risk-free" classroom climate in which external evaluation is minimized and errors are treated as a natural part of learning. In this kind of environment children can learn to monitor and evaluate their own efforts in relation to the goals they are trying to achieve. When external evaluation occurs, it takes the form of useful and specific feedback that assists the child's efforts toward the goal. Positive evaluation can focus on effort, improvement, and achievement of a standard, rather than on relative performance (Stipek, 1998). Corrective evaluation can take the form of specific suggestions for improvement, and children can be given an opportunity (and encouraged) to revise work to meet the standard. In addition, teachers can organize assignments so that children can see their progress and experience a sense of efficacy and control.

The types of assistance provided when children need help also affect mastery motivation and motivation for self-regulated performance. Assistance strategies should support what the child is trying to do in ways that preserve perceived competence and control and support future independent performance. Too much help can promote dependence rather than independent self-regulated learning (Nelson-Le Gall, 1992). Children can also learn how to find answers to their questions on their own, and classroom resources can be provided and arranged to support these efforts.

Peer assistance and support can be effective when the classroom climate encourages cooperative effort rather than competition. Primary school children may be embarrassed to ask for help from peers if they think this will reveal a lack of competence and encourage negative comparisons or judgments from others. Children can be encouraged to use peers, as well as adults, as resources and to work together on learning tasks or projects. These cooperative learning groups may support motivation and self-regulation more effectively when they grow out of children's common interests and spontaneous choices, rather than when their composition and goals are totally regulated by the teacher.

Table 9.1 summarizes the types of self-regulation that are developing during the primary school years and the major environmental influences that contribute to development.

SUMMARY

Primary school children have significantly greater self-regulatory capacities than younger children. They are also becoming consciously aware of their capabilities and are increasingly able to deliberately choose specific strategies to reach specific goals. Their growing awareness can lead to major advances in self-regulation, but it also makes this age group more vulnerable to assaults on their feelings of competence and control. Children of this age are beginning to compare themselves with others and to develop internal standards for achievement.

Children are also moving away from dependence on the family and adults in general during this period. They are increasingly interested in peer relationships and want to be accepted and effective in interactions with other children. Home and school environments that provide opportunities for children to interact positively and cooperatively with peers support the continued development of appropriate and effective strategies for controlling their own behavior and influencing others. As they move away from dependence on adults and develop internal standards for guiding behavior, primary school children become more vulnerable to peer standards and judgments. If the

TABLE 9.1. Developmental Milestones of Self-Regulation in Primary School Children and Major Environmental Supports

Domain of development	Milestones	Role of adults	Role of environment
Social/ emotional behavior	Capable of conscious self-control Can reliably abide by rules but may be rigid and punitive in applying them Capable of using language to regulate own behavior and influence others High peer interest and involvement—desire for acceptance makes peer norms more influential Capable of cooperative interaction with others: can engage in independent negotiation and social problem solving with peers and needs less direct adult supervision Can use problem-focused rather than emotion-focused strategies in interactions with others Can learn from discussions as well as direct experience Can play games with rules	Continue to function as models, resources, and guides, but emphasis now is on open and frequent communication with children about attitudes and values and issues that concern the child Can use guidance techniques that: • use problem-solving techniques • involve discussions about issues and problems (can now go beyond specific instances to general problems) • emphasize individual control/responsibility • involve general principles and standards • suggest appropriate strategies in context • bring decisions to conscious awareness Less need of direct supervision of all activities but importance of general adult monitoring of child's interests, peer influences, and involvement, media influences/involvement, and other activities outside family and school	Provides climate of respect, acceptance, and positive expectations for self-regulated behavior Contains opportunities for positive interactions with peers, both at home and at school Contains clear guidelines (appropriate for age and developmental level of the child or children) for responsibilities, opportunities (choices), expectations, and consequences, which are consistently and appropriately implemented Contains materials and activities that support constructive peer interaction Structured (classroom) experiences minimize exposure to negative behaviors and attitudes (that exist in the environment or culture), give attention to children's developmental level and ability to assimilate negative information, and include discussions with adults as well as peers when these exposures occur
Prosocial behavior	Can reflect on own and others' behaviors and their consequences Consciously aware that self and others have mental states and feelings Begins to understand the perspectives of others Interested in reciprocity and "fairness" Has some internalized standards of behavior and still developing others Shows somewhat stable prosocial (or antisocial) attitudes, values, and behaviors Can engage in conscious prosocial behaviors Has developed some degree of moral responsibility or "conscience" and is considered accountable for an increasing number of own actions	Model prosocial attitudes and behaviors Attribute prosocial motives to children Assign appropriate responsibilities to children Expect and encourage responsible behavior Monitor exposure to violent or antisocial models (live or media) and discuss behaviors or events that violate prosocial values with the child Guide the child away (when possible) from experiences that the adult believes would be harmful Provide guidelines for behavior that connect behavior with its effects and that include reference to general principles and values as well as the consequences of behaviors for others	Social climate and guidelines for behavior require, encourage, and support responsibility, respect, and care for others, and positive interaction styles and sanctions negative or antisocial behavior Provides opportunities for positive and cooperative interactions with others Includes materials and activities that encourage and support cooperative and prosocial behaviors and attitudes (board games, cooperative learning activities)

Cognitive self-regulation	Consciously aware of self and growing metacognitive awareness of own thinking processes—which increases the child's ability to consciously control and direct: • attention • memory and memory strategies • goal setting and choice of task or activity • overall planning and problem-solving activities • use of strategies in cognitive tasks • monitoring of ongoing activities—noticing progress and errors and correcting performance • sequencing activities in multistep tasks Can use private speech for reflection on alternatives and self-guidance in tasks Is developing internal standards for performance	Can teach self-regulatory strategies for use in cognitive tasks and problem solving, which include: • problem definition or goal setting • planning • strategy choice and implementation • response guidance or monitoring • self-reinforcement or evaluation Provide developmentally appropriate tasks and activities that include: • tasks and activities that are interesting to children • choices among appropriate alternatives • appropriate levels of challenge—not too easy or difficult for age and skill levels • ways for children to monitor, check, and correct their own work • opportunities for children to discover and create • the perception of control for the child Model and communicate effective language that can be incorporated in children's private speech for self-guidance Use scaffolding to broaden children's understanding and provide assistance (including suggesting appropriate task attack and problem-solving strategies in context)	Coherent but appropriately individualized expectations for performance or achievement Contains an appropriate range of challenging tasks and activities for every child's interests and abilities Provides enough flexibility for the child to have a reasonable amount of control over: • goals, tasks, and activities chosen • time spent in tasks and projects • criteria for evaluating outcomes Provides sufficient time for carrying out chosen and assigned activities (tasks are not rushed and there is time for reflection and self-correction) Contains sufficient space for performance of tasks and activities so that children are not distracted by crowding or constrained conditions Contains sufficient materials for carrying out tasks, projects, and other activities successfully
Motivation for self-regulation	Generalized need to feel competent is becoming differentiated to include specific areas of achievement Developing internal standards for performance and awareness of skills of others leads to increased self-judgment of own performance Needs to feel competent and able to control outcomes in order to want to engage in tasks in particular areas of competence	Demonstrate reinforcing attitudes toward independence, persistence, and self-regulated learning Design the environment for self-regulated learning with provision for responsible individual goal-setting, planning, and task accomplishment Be a resource, model, and guide rather than a dictator Design tasks and activities so that a child or small group can carry them out without constant adult direction Use evaluation techniques that reward self-regulated learning (vs. competition for external rewards, teacher attention, or being "first") Use assistance strategies that support what the child is trying to do and preserve perceived competence and control	Has a risk-free climate of respect for individual differences in interests, skills, and achievement Provides for a variety of interests, goals, and activities for children Includes flexible goals in different academic areas (allows for a range of abilities and interests and does not require that all children do the same thing at the same time) Provides appropriate level of challenges to match the child's interests and abilities Provides some materials that the child can structure independently Provides materials that the child can access and use independently

peer group models inappropriate or antisocial attitudes and behaviors, children are at greater risk of adopting them. However, ongoing positive and trusting relationships with adults can reduce the effects of negative peer influences. These relationships, as well as positive cooperative experiences with peers, can also preserve and strengthen prosocial dispositions in children.

The early elementary years provide both opportunities and risks for developing cognitive self-regulation. The challenges presented by formal schooling can lead to real and perceived increases in competence and control. They can also lead to perceived failure or helplessness and a reduced willingness to attempt self-direction. When teachers allow children to choose among interesting and appropriately challenging alternatives and provide feedback or assistance in ways that support independent effort and perceived control, children are more interested in cognitive activities, invest more energy in pursuing them, and take more responsibility for the outcomes.

Support for cognitive self-regulation can now include both strategy training and deliberate efforts to bring children's self-regulatory capacities to their conscious awareness. Teaching techniques based on behavioral, social learning, and Vygotskian theory have been proposed. Their relative usefulness can be considered in relation to children's maturity and capacity for "constructive" and symbolic processing. Generally, strategy training should support children's independent efforts and their perception of competence and control.

As children become more aware of themselves and of external standards for evaluating their performance, their motivation for mastery and for self-regulatory control is affected by how they evaluate their capacities and their products. Children who believe they are competent attempt more challenging tasks and are more interested in personal responsibility and control. Children who experience failure, or believe that goals and outcomes are controlled by others, are less motivated to put forth effort, regulate their own activities, or care about the outcome. Teaching methods that emphasize external control (with inflexible goals and reliance on external rewards and punishments), use uncontrollable evaluation criteria (evaluating children by comparison with others, expecting them to meet unrealistic standards, or using criteria they cannot understand), or employ assistance strategies that reduce feelings of control (by overdirection or an emphasis on "right answers" rather than strategies that can be used independently) undermine and diminish children's belief in themselves and their willingness to try. Teaching methods that emphasize internal control (by providing choice and support for individual ideas and performance styles), use controllable evaluation criteria (such as emphasizing effort and improvement, viewing error as an opportunity for learning, and allowing repeated efforts to meet performance criteria), and provide assistance strategies that preserve feelings of control and competence (by scaffolding children's own efforts and suggesting strategies that will support these efforts) increase children's belief in their competence and ability to control and direct their own learning.

Epilogue

The chapters in this book discuss a variety of theoretical and research perspectives on the nature and nurture of self-regulation in young children and suggest applications for practice that are based on this work. With the exception of Vygotsky's theory, which focuses on the importance of cultural context, all of the theories reflect western European values and assumptions. Although an increasing amount of cross-cultural research is now being carried out, most of the research related to the development of self-regulation has been done with western European parents, teachers, schools, and children.

The definitions of self-regulation provided by this body of work, the value placed on self-direction and control, and the suggested social, cognitive, and motivational outcomes proposed as goals for development are also influenced, if not determined, by the value structure of the Western cultural tradition. This is a tradition that values independent effort and achievement, self-reliance, and personal responsibility. Other cultural traditions may place a lower value on these goals or may consider them to be negative outcomes. Even within the Western tradition some countries focus more on aesthetic and social development than is the case in the United States.

The brain structures available to support executive functioning are universal, but the strength, direction, and goals for control are provided by experience. The interconnections between neurons that survive and thrive are determined to a large extent by experience, and cultural factors determine what these experiences will be. Primary goals for control might be conformity with others, preserving established ways of behaving and thinking, establishing dominance over others, or any number of other possibilities. Additional research is needed to understand the forms of self-regulation that other cultural groups value and how these may be supported in development.

This book also raises issues related to child-rearing practice in the United States. It emphasizes the critical importance of the early years and the central role(s) played by a child's primary caregiver(s) in the development of self-regulation. Close, trusting relationships between adults and children are strongly linked to the development of emotional control and positive social behaviors. Given the importance of such development for the common culture, it is interesting that professional or "job" training is considered more important than training for the job of parenting. Better educated parents often turn to "how to" books for advice about child raising or discipline, and "high risk" parents may receive special training as part of early intervention programs, but the society as a whole has not focused on these issues. In a diverse culture research cannot tell parents what to teach children, but it can help them understand the probable effects of different child-rearing methods.

As children spend less time with parents and more time in alternate forms of care, the quality of that care becomes a focus of concern for society. If children need warm, responsive, and consistent care by primary caregivers who attend to their individuality, and environments that provide coherence and appropriate levels of stimulation and challenge, the cost of alternate care will be great. Minimal educational requirements and low pay for child care workers (currently leading to high turnover rates in child care centers) will not lead to high-quality care. Society may not be ready to accept the cost of high-quality care, but an alternate question is whether society is ready to accept the outcomes of low-quality care.

Finally, issues raised in this book also have implications for educational practice in schools. In early education there is a consensus that young children are learning to be independent—to control and direct their behavior effectively both in interaction with others and when engaged in mastery tasks. There is an understanding that young children function in an integrated way and a traditional value for teaching the "whole child." Teachers of young children know that they learn about the world and learn to solve problems when they play and that play is their way of experimenting with new ideas and practicing skills. When adults love their "work," much of it is also "play" for them. Early childhood educators need to hold fast to these understandings in the face of increasing "academic standards" for early childhood classrooms. It is not that young children cannot or should not learn letters and numbers and concepts in science, because they can and are interested in these concepts if presented appropriately. However, long periods of teacher instruction and longer periods of filling out work sheets at desks or tables are not the most effective means of supporting learning, self-regulated learning, or love of learning at these ages.

In later schooling the recommended shift in focus, from imparting knowledge to fostering self-regulated learning, although suggested by both theory and research, is especially difficult to accomplish and can generate controversy. It is difficult to accomplish because teachers have to be trained to implement self-regulated learning and must believe it to be beneficial. It can generate controversy because parents, teachers, administrators, and public policy makers may fail to understand or disagree with its methods and goals. In a climate that emphasizes "basic" academic skills and short-term accountability, it is harder to focus on skills that will serve a lifetime and long-term (life outcomes) accountability. It is also easier to test a child's knowledge of specific subject matter than whether that child is acquiring the skills and motivation to be a lifelong learner and the judgment and internal control to regulate her life effectively.

In our complex culture children certainly need to be literate and to understand mathematics and science and history, but they also need to become "educated" in a way that makes them value learning and believe that they can be competent learners. If children come to see knowledge as "cultural tools" that will enable them to experience life more deeply and direct their lives more effectively and successfully, becoming educated can become an internal and chosen goal. Schools can support this understanding by building appropriate choice and individual control into a curriculum that interests and challenges each individual at an appropriate level, emphasizes internal rewards rather than external control, and allows space and time for each child's personal quest.

References

Achenbach, T. M., & Edelbrock, C. (1981). Behavioral problems and competencies of normal and disturbed children aged four to sixteen. *Monographs of the Society for Research in Child Development, 46*(1, Serial No. 188).

Achenbach, T. M., & Edelbrock, C. (1991). National survey of the problems and competencies among four-to sixteen-year-olds. *Monographs of the Society for Research in Child Development, 56*(3, Serial No. 225).

Adler, A. (1956). *The individual psychology of Alfred Adler: A systematic presentation of selections from his writings* (H. L. Ansbacher & R. R. Ansbacher, Eds.). New York: Basic Books.

Ainsworth, M. D. S., & Bell, S. M. (1972). Mother-infant interaction and the development of competence. In K. J. Connolly & J. S. Bruner (Eds.), *The growth of competence.* New York: Academic Press.

Ainsworth, M. D. S., Bell, S. M., & Stayton, D. J. (1972). Individual differences in the development of some attachment behaviors. *Merrill-Palmer Quarterly of Behavior and Development, 18,* 123–142.

Ainsworth, M. D. S., Bell, S., & Stayton, D. (1974). Infant-mother attachment and social development: Socialization as a product of reciprocal responsiveness to signals. In M. Richards (Ed.), *The integration of the child into the social world.* Cambridge, UK: Cambridge University Press.

Alexander, K. L., & Entwisle, D. R. (1988). Achievement in the first two years of school: Patterns and processes. *Monographs of the Society for Research in Child Development, 53*(2, Serial No. 218).

Als, H. (1978). Assessing an assessment: Conceptual considerations, methodological issues, and a perspective on the future of the Neonatal Behavioral Assessment Scale. In A. J. Sameroff (Ed.), Organization and stability: A commentary on the Brazelton Neonatal Behavioral Assessment Scale. *Monographs of the Society for Research in Child Development, 43*(5–6, Serial No. 177).

Als, H., & Gilkerson, L. (1995, June/July). Developmentally supportive care in the neonatal intensive care unit. *Zero to Three,* pp. 2–9.

Als, H., Lawhon, G., McAnulty, G. B., Gibes-Grosman, R., & Blickman, J. G. (1994). Individualized developmental care for the very low-birth-weight preterm infant: Medical and neurological effects. *Journal of the American Medical Association, 272,* 853–891.

Ames, L. B., & Ilg, F. L. (1976). *Your two-year-old.* New York: Dell.

Ames, L. B., Ilg, F. L., & Haber, C. C. (1982). *Your one-year-old.* New York: Dell.

American Psychological Association. (1993). *Learner-centered psychological principles: Guidelines for school redesign and reform.* Washington, DC: Author.

Arsenio, W., & Cooperman, S. (1996). Children's conflict-related emotions: Implications for morality and autonomy. In M. Killen (Ed.), *New directions for child development: No. 73. Children's autonomy, social competence, and interactions with adults and other children: Exploring connections and consequences.* San Francisco: Jossey-Bass.

Asendorpf, J. (1989). Individual, differential, and aggregate stability of social competence. In B. Schneider, G. Attili, J. Nadel, & R. Weissberg (Eds.), *Social competence in developmental perspective.* Boston: Klewer Academic.

Asher, S. R., & Dodge, K. A. (1986). Identifying children who are rejected by their peers. *Developmental Psychology, 22,* 444–449.

Asher, S. R., & Renshaw, P. D. (1981). Children without friends: Social knowledge and social skills training. In S. Asher, & J. Gottman (Eds.), *The development of children's friendships.* New York: Cambridge University Press.

Asher, S. R., & Wheeler, V. A. (1985). Children's loneliness: A comparison of rejected and neglected peer states. *Journal of Counseling and Clinical Psychology, 53,* 500–505.

Ashman, A. F., & Das, J. P. (1980). Relationship between planning and simultaneous-successive processing. *Perceptual and Motor Skills, 51,* 371–382.

Astington, J. W., & Olson, D. R. (1995). The cognitive revolution in children's understanding of mind. *Human Development, 38,* 179–189.

Atkinson, J. W. (1957). Motivational determinants of risk taking behavior. *Psychological Review, 64,* 359–372.

Baddeley, A. (1986). *Working memory*. Oxford, UK: Oxford University Press.

Baddeley, A. Della Salla, S., Gray, C., Papagno, C., & Spinnler, H. (1997). Testing central executive functioning with a paper-and-pencil test. In P. Rabbitt (Ed.), *Methodology of frontal and executive functions*. East Sussex, UK: Psychology Press.

Baker, L. (1989). Metacognition, comprehension monitoring, and the adult reader. *Educational Psychology Review, 1,* 3–38.

Baker, L., & Brown, A. L. (1984). Metacognitive skills and reading. In P. D. Pearson (Ed.), *Handbook of reading research*. New York: Longman.

Baker-Sennett, J., Matusov, E., & Rogoff, B. (1993). Sociocultural processes of creative planning in children's playcrafting. In P. Light, & G. Butterworth (Eds.), *Context and cognition: Ways of learning and knowing*. Hillsdale, NJ: Erlbaum.

Baldwin, D. A., & Moses, L. J. (1996). The ontogeny of social information gathering. *Child Development, 67,* 1915–1939.

Baldwin, J. D., & Baldwin, J. I. (1998). *Behavior principles in everyday life*. Upper Saddle River, NJ: Prentice-Hall.

Bandura, A. (1973). *Aggression: A social learning analysis*. Englewood Cliffs, NJ: Prentice-Hall.

Bandura, A. (1977). *Social learning theory*. Englewood Cliffs, NJ: Prentice-Hall.

Bandura, A. (1978). The self-system in reciprocal determinism. *American Psychologist, 33,* 344–358.

Bandura, A. (1982). Self efficacy mechanism in human agency. *American Psychologist, 37,* 122–147.

Bandura, A. (1986). *Social foundations of thought and action: A social cognitive theory*. Englewood Cliffs, NJ: Prentice-Hall.

Bandura, A. (1997). *Self-efficacy: The exercise of control*. New York: Freeman.

Bandura, A., Ross, D., & Ross, S. A. (1963). Imitation of film-mediated aggressive models. *Journal of Abnormal and Social Psychology, 66,* 3–11.

Barkley, R. A. (1997). *ADHD and the nature of self-control*. New York: Guilford Press.

Barkley, R. A. (1998). *Attention-deficit hyperactivity disorder: A handbook for diagnosis and treatment* (2nd ed.). New York: Guilford Press.

Bartlett, F. C. (1932). *Remembering: A study in experimental and social psychology*. Cambridge, UK: Cambridge University Press.

Bauer, P. J., Schwade, J. A., Wewerka, S. S., & Delaney, K. (1999). Planning ahead: Goal-directed problem solving by 2-year-olds. *Developmental Psychology, 35,* 1321–1337.

Baumrind, D. (1967). Child care practices anteceding three patterns of preschool behavior. *Genetic Psychology Monographs, 75,* 43–88.

Baumrind, D. (1971). Current patterns of parental authority. *Developmental Psychology Monographs, 4,* 1–103.

Baumrind, D. (1973). The development of instrumental competence through socialization. In A. Pick (Ed.), *Minnesota Symposia on Child Psychology* (Vol. 7). Minneapolis: University of Minnesota Press.

Bereiter, C., & Scardamalia, M. (1986). Educational relevance of the study of expertise. *Interchange, 17,* 10–17.

Berk, L. E. (1992). Children's private speech: An overview of theory and the status of research. In R. M. Diaz & L. E. Berk (Eds.), *Private speech: From social interaction to self-regulation.* Hillsdale, NJ: Erlbaum.

Berk, L. E. (1994, November). Why children talk to themselves. *Scientific American, 271,* 78–83.

Berk, L. E., & Winsler, A. (1995). *Scaffolding children's learning: Vygotsky and early childhood education.* Washington, DC: National Association for the Education of Young Children.

Berkowitz, M. W. (1982). Self-control development and relation to prosocial behavior: A response to Peterson. *Merrill-Palmer Quarterly, 28,* 223–236.

Berlyne, D. E. (1960). *Conflict, arousal and curiosity.* New York: McGraw-Hill.

Berlyne, D. E. (1969). Laughter, humor and play. In G. Lindzey & E. Aronson (Eds.), *Handbook of social psychology* (2nd ed., Vol. 3). Reading, MA: Addison-Wesley.

Berrueta-Clement, J. R., Schweinhart, L. J., Barnett, W. S., Epstein, A. S., & Weikart, D. P. (1984). *Changed lives: The effects of the Perry Preschool Program on youths through age 19.* Ypsilanti, MI: High/Scope Press.

Bickhard, M. H. (1990). Scaffolding and self-scaffolding: Critical aspects of development. In L. T. Winigar & J. Valsiner (Eds.), *Children's development within social context: Vol. 1. Metatheory and theory.* Hillsdale, NJ: Erlbaum.

Bidell, T. R., & Fischer, K. W. (1994). Developmental transitions in children's early on-line planning. In M. Haith, R. Roberts, J. Benson, & B. Pennington (Eds.), *The development of future oriented processes.* Chicago: University of Chicago Press.

Biemiller, A., & Meichenbaum, D. (1992). A perspective on cognitive research and its implications for instruction. In L. B. Resnick & L. E. Klopfer (Eds.), *Toward the thinking curriculum: Current cognitive research.* Alexandria, VA: Association for Supervision and Curriculum Development.

Biemiller, A., & Meichenbaum, D. (1998). *Nurturing independent learners:*

Helping students take charge of their learning. Cambridge, MA: Brookline Books.

Bjorklund, D. F. (1990). *Children's strategies: Contemporary views of cognitive development.* Hillsdale, NJ: Erlbaum.

Block, J. H., & Block, J. (1980). The role of ego-control and ego-resilience in the organization of behavior. In W. Andrew Collins (Ed.). *Minnesota Symposia on Child Psychology: Vol. 13. Development of cognition, affect, and social relations.* Minneapolis: University of Minnesota Press.

Borkowski, J. G. (1992). Metacognitive theory: A framework for teaching literacy, writing, and math skills. *Journal of Learning Disabilities, 25,* 253–257.

Bower, T. G. R. (1977). *A primer of infant development.* San Francisco: W. H, Freeman.

Bowman, B. T., & Svetina, D. (1992). Social/emotional readiness. In *National Education Goals Report: Building a nation of learners.* Washington, DC: U.S. Government Printing Office.

Brazelton, T. B. (1978). Introduction. In A. J. Sameroff (Ed.), Organization and stability: A commentary on the Brazelton Neonatal Behavior Assessment Scale. *Monographs of the Society for Research in Child Development, 43* (5–6, Serial No. 177).

Breger, L. (1973). *From instinct to identity.* Englewood Cliffs, NJ: Prentice-Hall.

Brenner, E. M., & Salovey, P. (1997). Emotion regulation during childhood: Developmental, interpersonal, and individual considerations. In P. Salovey & D. Slayter (Eds.), *Emotional development and emotional intelligence: Educational implications.* New York: Basic Books.

Brickman, P., Rabinowitz, V. C., Karuza, J., Coates, D., Cohn, E., & Kidder, L. (1982). Models of helping and coping. *American Psychologist, 37,* 368–384.

Bronfenbrenner, U. (1990). Who cares for children? *Research and Clinical Center for Child Development, 12,* 27–40.

Bronowski, J. (1977). Human and animal languages. In *A sense of the future.* Cambridge, MA: MIT Press. (Reprinted from 1967, *To honor Roman Jakobson* [Vol. 1]. The Hague, Netherlands: Mouton).

Bronson, M. B. (1985). *Manual for the Bronson Social and Task Skill Profile.* Chestnut Hill, MA: Boston College.

Bronson, M. B. (1994). The usefulness of an observational measure of children's social and mastery behaviors in early childhood classrooms. *Early Childhood Research Quarterly, 9,* 19–43.

Bronson, M. B. (1995). *The right stuff for children birth to 8: Selecting play materials to support development.* Washington, DC: National Association for the Education of Young Children.

Bronson, M. B., Pierson, D. E., & Tivnan, T. (1984). The effects of early education on children's competence in elementary school. *Evaluation Review, 8,* 615–629.

Bronson, W. C. (1973, March). *Mother–toddler interaction: A perspective on studying the development of competence.* Paper presented at the Merrill-Palmer Conference on Research and Teaching of Infant Development, Detroit, MI.

Brown, A. L. (1978). Knowing when, where, and how to remember: A problem in metacognition. In R. Glaser (Ed.), *Advances in instructional psychology* (Vol. 1). Hillsdale, NJ: Erlbaum.

Brown, A. L. (1982). Learning and development: The problems of compatibility, access, and induction. *Human Development, 25,* 89–115.

Brown, A. L., Bransford, J. D., Ferrera, R. A., & Campione, J. C. (1983). Learning, remembering and understanding. In J. Flavell & E. Mankman (Eds.), *Carmichael's manual of child psychology* (Vol. 1). New York: Wiley.

Brown, A. L., & Campione, J. (1981). Inducing flexible thinking: A problem of access. In M. Friedman, J. Das, & N. O'Connor (Eds.), *Intelligence and learning.* New York: Plenum.

Brown, A. L., & DeLoache, J. S. (1978). Skills, plans, and self-regulation. In R. S. Siegler (Ed.), *Children's thinking: What develops?* Hillsdale, NJ: Erlbaum.

Brown, R. A. (1973). *A first language, the early stage.* Cambridge, MA: Harvard University Press.

Bruner, J. S. (1968). *Processes of cognitive growth in infancy.* Heinz Werner Lectures, Clark University, Worcester, MA.

Bruner, J. S. (1969a). Processes of growth in infancy. In A. Ambrose (Ed.), *Stimulation in early infancy.* London: Academic Press.

Bruner, J. B. (1969b, July). *Origins of problem solving strategies in skill acquisition.* Paper presented at the 19th International Congress of Psychology, London.

Bruner, J. S. (1970). The growth and structure of skill. In K. J. Connolly (Ed.), *Mechanisms of motor skill development.* New York: Academic Press.

Bruner, J. S. (1972). The nature and uses of immaturity. *American Psychologist, 27,* 1–22.

Bruner, J. S. (1986). *Actual minds, possible worlds.* Cambridge, MA: Harvard University Press.

Bruner, J. S. (1990). *Acts of meaning.* Cambridge, MA: Harvard University Press.

Canfield, R. L., Smith, E. G., Brezsnyak, M. P., & Snow, K. L. (1997). Information processing through the first year of life: A longitudinal study using the visual expectation paradigm. *Monographs of the Society for Research in Child Development, 62*(2, Serial No. 250).

Caplan, F., & Caplan, T. (1977). *The second twelve months of life.* Toronto: Bantam Books.

Carlson, M., & Earls, F. (1998). Psychological and neuroendocrinological sequelae of early social deprivation in institutionalized children in Romania. In *Integrative neurobiology of affiliation.* New York: Academy of Science.

Case, R. (1985). *Intellectual development: Birth to adulthood.* Orlando, FL: Academic Press.

Case, R. (1992). The role of the frontal lobes in the regulation of cognitive behavior. *Brain and Cognition, 20,* 51–73.

Casey, M. B., Bronson, M. B., Tivnan, T., Riley, E., & Spenciner, L. (1991). Differentiating preschoolers' sequential planning ability from their general intelligence: A study of organization. *Journal of Applied Developmental Psychology, 12,* 19–31.

Casey, M. B., & Lippman, M. (1991). Learning to plan through play. *Young Children, 46,* 52–58.

Casey, M. B., & Tucker, E. C. (1994, October). Lifelong learning in a problem-centered classroom. *Phi Delta Kappan,* 139–143.

Caspi, A. (1998). Personality development across the life span. In N. Eisenberg (Ed.), W. Damon (Series Ed.), *Handbook of child psychology: Vol. 3. Social, emotional, and personality development* (5th ed.). New York: Wiley.

Cavanaugh, J. C., & Perlmutter, M. (1982). Metamemory: A critical examination. *Child Development, 53,* 11–28.

Chandler, M. J. (1973). Egocentrism and antisocial behavior; The assessment and training of social perspective taking skills. *Developmental Psychology, 9,* 326–332.

Changeux, J. P., & Dehaene, S. (1993). Neuronal models of cognitive functions. In M. H. Johnson (Ed.), *Brain development and cognition: A reader.* Oxford, UK: Blackwell.

Chugani, H. T. (1997). Neuroimaging of developmental non-linearity and developmental pathologies. In R. W. Thatcher, G. R. Lyon, J. Rumsey, & N. Krasnegor (Eds.), *Developmental neuroimaging: Mapping the development of brain and behavior.* San Diego: Academic Press.

Chugani, H. T., Phelps, M. E., & Mazziotta, J. C. (1993). Positron emission tomography study of human brain functional development. In M. H. Johnson (Ed.), *Brain development and cognition: A reader.* Oxford, UK: Blackwell.

Cirino, R. J., & Beck, S. J. (1991). Social information processing and the effects of reputational, situational, developmental and gender factors among children's sociometric groups. *Merrill-Palmer Quarterly, 37,* 561–582.

Clarke-Stewart, A., Gruber, C. P., & Fitzgerald, L. M. (1994). *Children at home and in day care.* Hillsdale, NJ: Erlbaum.

Cocking, R. R., & Copple, C. E. (1987). Social influences on representational awareness: Plans for representing and plans as representation. In S. L. Friedman, E. K. Scholnick, & R. R. Cocking (Eds.), *Blueprints for thinking: The role of planning in cognitive development.* Cambridge, UK: Cambridge University Press.

Coie, J. D., & Dodge, K. A. (1983). Continuities and changes in children's social status: A five-year longitudinal study. *Merrill-Palmer Quarterly, 29,* 261–282.

Cole, M. (1990). Cognitive development and formal schooling: The evidence from cross-cultural research. In L. C. Moll (Ed.), *Vygotsky and education.* Cambridge, UK: Cambridge University Press.

Cole, M. (1992). Culture in development. In M. Bornstein & M. Lamb (Eds.), *Developmental psychology: An advanced textbook* (3rd ed.). Hillsdale, NJ: Erlbaum.

Cole, M., Gay, J., Glick, J. A., & Sharp, D. W. (1971). *The cultural context of learning and thinking.* New York: Basic Books.

Cole, M., & Scribner, S. (1974). *Culture and thought: A psychological introduction.* New York: Wiley.

Cole, P., Barrett, K., & Zahn-Waxler, C. (1992). Emotional displays in two-year-olds during mishaps. *Child Development, 63,* 314–324.

Compas, B. E. (1987). Coping with stress during childhood and adolescence. *Psychological Bulletin, 101,* 393–403.

Condry, J., & Siman, M. L. (1974). Characteristics of peer- and adult-oriented children. *Journal of Marriage and the Family, 36,* 543–554.

Cooper, J., & Fazio, R. H. (1984). A new look at dissonance theory. *Advances in Experimental and Social Psychology* (Vol. 17). New York: Academic Press.

Corno, L. (1992). Encouraging students to take responsibility for learning and performance. *Elementary School Journal, 93,* 69–83.

Corrigan, R., & Denton, P. (1996). Causal understanding as a developmental primitive. *Developmental Review, 16,* 162–202.

Crick, N. R., & Ladd, G. W. (1990). Children's perceptions of the outcomes of social strategies: Do the ends justify the means? *Developmental Psychology, 26,* 612–620.

Crockenberg, S., Jackson, S., & Langrock, A. M. (1996). Autonomy and goal attainment: Parenting, gender and children's social competence. In M. Killen (Ed.), *New directions for child development: No. 73. Children's Autonomy, social competence, and interactions with adults and other children: Exploring connections and consequences.* San Francisco: Jossey-Bass.

Cummings, E. M., Hennessy, K. D., & Sugarman, D. B. (1994). Responses of physically abused boys to interadult anger involving their mothers. *Development and Psychopathology, 6,* 31–41.

Cummings, E. M., Simpson, K. S., & Wilson, A. (1993). Children's responses to interadult anger as a function of information about resolution. *Developmental Psychology, 29,* 978–985.

Cummings, E. M., Zahn-Waxler, C., & Radke-Yarrow, M. (1984). Developmental changes in children's reactions to anger in the home. *Journal of Child Psychology and Psychiatry, 25,* 63–74.

Cummings, J. L. (1995). Anatomic and behavioral aspects of frontal-subcortical circuits. In J. Grafman, K. J. Holyoak, & F. Boller (Eds.), *Structure and functions of the human prefrontal cortex: Vol. 769. Annals of the New York Academy of Sciences.* New York: New York Academy of Sciences.

Damasio, A. (1994). *Descartes's error: Emotion, reason and the human brain.* New York: Grosset/Putnam.

Damon, W., & Hart, D. (1988). *Self understanding from childhood and adolescence.* New York: Cambridge University Press.

Das, J. P. (1980). Planning: Theoretical considerations and empirical evidence. *Psychological Research, 41,* 141–151.

Das, J. P. (1984). Aspects of planning. In J. R. Kirby (Ed.), *Cognitive strategies and educational performance.* New York: Academic Press.

Dawson, G., Hessl, D., & Frey, K. (1994). Social influences on early developing biological and behavioral systems related at risk for affective disorder. In *Development and psychopathology.* Cambridge, UK: Cambridge University Press.

deCharms, R. (1968). *Personal causation.* New York: Academic Press.

deCharms, R. (1971). From pawns to origins: Toward self-motivation. In G. S. Lesser (Ed.), *Psychology and educational practice.* Glenview, NJ: Scott, Foresman.

deCharms, R. (1976). *Enhancing motivation: Change in the classroom.* New York: Irvington.

deCharms, R. (1984). Motivation enhancement in educational settings. In R. Ames & C. Ames (Eds.), *Research on motivation in education: Vol. 1. Student motivation.* San Diego, CA: Academic Press.

Deci, E. L. (1980). *The psychology of self-determination.* Lexington, MA: Heath.

Deci, E. L., & Porak, J. (1978). Cognitive evaluation theory and the study of human motivation. In M. R. Lepper & D. Green (Eds.), *The hidden costs of reward: New perspectives on the psychology of human motivation.* Hillsdale, NJ: Erlbaum.

Deci, E. L., & Ryan, R. M. (1985). *Intrinsic motivation and self-determina-tion in human behavior.* New York: Plenum.

Deci, E. L., & Ryan, R. M. (1987). The support of autonomy and the con-trol of behavior. *Journal of Personality and Social Psychology, 53,* 1024–1037.

Deci, E. L., & Ryan, R. M. (1991). A motivational approach to self: Integra-tion in personality. In R. A. Dienstbier (Ed.), *Nebraska Symposium on Motivation 1990* (Vol. 38). Lincoln: University of Nebraska Press.

DeLisi, R. (1987). A cognitive–developmental model of planning. In S. L. Friedman, E. K. Scholnick & R. R. Cocking (Eds.), *Blueprints for thinking: The role of planning in cognitive development.* Cambridge, UK: Cambridge University Press.

DeLoach, J. S., & Brown, A. L. (1987). The early emergence of planning skills in children. In J. Bruner & H. Haste (Eds.), *Making sense: The child's construction of the world.* London: Methuen.

Denckla, M. B., & Reader, M. J. (1993). Education and psychosocial inter-ventions: Executive dysfunction and its consequences. In R. Kurlan (Ed.), *Handbook of Tourette's Syndrome and related tic and behavioral disorders.* New York: Marcel Dekker.

Denham, S. A., Mason, R., & Couchoud, E. A. (1995). Scaffolding young children's prosocial responsiveness: Preschoolers' responses to adult sadness, anger, and pain. *International Journal of Behavioral Develop-ment, 18,* 489–504.

Denham, S. A., Mitchell-Copeland, J., Strandberg, K., Blair, K., & Auer-bach, S. (1997). Parent contributions to preschoolers' emotional com-petence: Direct and indirect effects. *Motivation and Emotion, 21,* 65–86.

Dennis, M. (1991). Frontal lobe function in childhood and adolescence: A heuristic for assessing attention regulation, executive control, and the intentional states important for social discourse. *Developmental Neu-ropsychology, 7,* 327–358.

Derryberry, D., & Rothbart, M. K. (1988). Arousal, affect, and attention as components of temperament. *Journal of Personality and Social Psy-chology, 55,* 958–966.

Devereux, E. C. (1970). The role of peer-group experience in moral develop-ment. In J. P. Hill (Ed.), *Minnesota Symposia on Child Psychology* (Vol. 4). Minneapolis: University of Minnesota Press.

Diamond, K. E. (1993). Factors in preschool children's social problem-solv-ing strategies for peers with and without disabilities. *Early Childhood Research Quarterly, 9,* 195–205.

Diamond, M. C. (1988). *Enriching heredity: The impact of the environment on the anatomy of the brain.* New York: Free Press.

Diener, C. I., & Dweck, C. S. (1978). An analysis of learned helplessness: Continuous changes in performance, strategy, and achievement cognitions following failure. *Journal of Personality and Social Psychology, 36,* 451–462.

Dix, T. (1991). The affective organization of parenting: Adaptive and maladaptive processes. *Psychological Bulletin, 110,* 3–25.

Dodge, K. A. (1983). Behavioral antecedents of peer social status. *Child Development, 54,* 1386–1399.

Dodge, K. A. (1985). Facets of social interaction and the assessment of social competence in children. In B. Schneider, K. Rubin, & J. Ledingham (Eds.), *Children's peer relations: Issues in assessment and intervention.* New York: Springer-Verlag.

Dodge, K. A. (1986). A social information processing model of social competence in children. In M. Perlmutter (Ed.), *Minnesota Symposium on Child Psychology, 25,* 339–342.

Dodge, K. A., & Coie, J. D. (1987). Social information-processing factors in reactive and proactive aggression in children's peer groups. *Journal of Personality and Social Psychology, 53,* 1146–1158.

Dodge, K. A., Pettit, G. S., McClasky, C. L., & Brown, M. M. (1986). Social competence in children. *Monographs of the Society for Research in Child Development, 51*(2, Serial No. 213).

Doise, W. (1990). The development of individual competencies through social interaction. In H. Foot, M. Morgan, & R. Sure (Eds.), *Children helping children.* New York: Wiley.

Dollard, J. Doob, L. W., Miller, N. E., Mowrer, D. H., & Sears, R. R. (1939). *Frustration and aggression.* New Haven, CT: Yale University Press.

Dollard, J., & Miller, N. E. (1941). *Social learning and imitation.* New Haven, CT: Yale University Press.

Dollard, J., & Miller, N. E. (1950). *Personality and psychotherapy? An analysis in terms of learning, thinking, and culture.* New York: McGraw-Hill.

Donaldson, M. (1978). *Children's minds.* New York: Norton.

Donaldson, M. (1987). The origins of inference. In J. Bruner & H. Haste (Eds.), *Making sense: The child's construction of the world.* London: Methuen.

Downey, G., & Coyne, J. C. (1990). Children of depressed parents: An integrative review. *Psychological Bulletin, 108,* 30–76.

Duell, O. K. (1986). Metacognitive skills. In G. D. Phye & T. Andre (Eds.), *Cognitive classroom learning: Understanding, thinking, and problem solving.* Orlando: Academic Press.

Dumas, J. E., & LaFreniere, P. J. (1993). Mother–child relationships as sources of support or stress: A comparison of competent, average, aggressive and anxious dyads. *Child Development, 64,* 1732–1754.

Dunn, J. (1988). *The beginnings of social understanding.* Cambridge, MA: Harvard University Press.

Dunn, J. (1996). The Emanuel Miller Memorial Lecture 1995: Children's relationships: Bridging the divide between cognitive and social development. *Journal of Child Psychology and Psychiatry and Allied Disciplines, 37,* 507–518.

Dunn, J., & Munn, P. (1986). Siblings and the development of prosocial behaviors. *International Journal of Behavioral Development, 9,* 265–284.

Dweck, C. S. (1975). The role of expectations and attributions in the alleviation of learned helplessness. *Journal of Personality and Social Psychology, 31,* 674–685.

Dweck, C. S. (1986). Motivational processes affecting learning. *American Psychologist, 41,* 1040–1048

Dweck, C. S. (1991). Self-theories and goals: Their role in motivation, personality, and development. In R. A. Dienstbier (Ed.), *Nebraska Symposium on Motivation: Vol. 38. Perspectives on motivation.* Lincoln: University of Nebraska Press.

Dweck, C. S., & Elliott, E. S. (1983). Achievement motivation. In O. M. Hetherington (Ed.), *Handbook of child psychology: Vol. 4. Socialization, personality, and social development.* New York: Wiley.

Dweck, C. S., & Goetz, T. (1978). Attribution and learned helplessness. In W. Harvey & R. Kidd (Eds.), *New directions in attribution research* (Vol. 2). Hillsdale, NJ: Erlbaum.

Dweck, C. S., & Repucci, N. (1973). Learned helplessness and reinforcement responsibility in children. *Journal of Personality and Social Psychology, 25,* 109–116.

Edelman, G. M. (1987). *Neural Darwinism.* New York: Basic Books.

Edelman, G. M. (1992). *Bright air, brilliant fire: On the matter of the mind.* New York: Basic Books.

Egeland, B., Carlson, E., & Sroufe, L. A. (1993). Resilience as process. In *Development and psychopathology.* Cambridge, UK: Cambridge University Press.

Eibl-Eibesfeldt, I. (1970). *Ethology: The biology of behavior.* New York: Holt, Rinehart and Winston.

Eisenberg, N., Cameron, E., Tryon, K., & Dodez, R. (1981). Socialization of prosocial behavior in preschool children. *Developmental Psychology, 17,* 773–782.

Eisenberg, N., & Fabes, R. A. (1992). Emotion, regulation, and the development of social competence. In M. S. Clark (Ed.), *Review of personality and social psychology: Vol. 14. Emotion and social behavior.* Newbury Park, CA: Sage.

Eisenberg, N., Fabes, R. A., Bernzweig, J., Karbon, M., Poulin, R., & Hanish, L. (1993). The relations of emotionality and regulation to preschoolers' social skills and sociometric status. *Child Development, 64,* 1418–1438.

Eisenberg, N., Fabes, R. A., Guthrie, I. K., Murphy, B. C., Maszk, P., Holmgren, R., & Suh, K. (1996). The relations of regulation and emotionality to problem behavior in elementary school children. *Development and Psychopathology, 8,* 141–162.

Eisenberg, N., Fabes, R. A., & Losoya, S. (1997). Emotional responding: Regulation, social correlates, and socialization. In P. Salovey & D. Sluyter (Eds.), *Emotional development and emotional intelligence: Educational implications.* New York: Basic Books.

Eisenberg, N., Fabes, R. A., Murphy, B., Maszk, P., Smith, M., & Karbon, M. (1995). The role of emotionality and regulation in children's social functioning: A longitudinal study. *Child Development, 66,* 1360–1384.

Eisenberg, N., Fabes, R. A., Schaller, M., Carlo, G., & Miller, P. (1991). The relations of parental characteristics and practices to children's vicarious emotional responding. *Child Development, 62,* 1393–1408.

Eisenberg, N., Fabes, R. A., Shepard, S. A., Murphy, B. C., Guthrie, I. K., Jones, S., Friedman, J., Poulin, R., & Maszk, P. (1997). Contemporaneous and longitudinal prediction of children's social functioning from regulation and emotionality. *Child Development, 68,* 642–664.

Eisenberg, N., Guthrie, I. K., Fabes, R. A., Reiser, M., Murphy, B. C., Holgren, R., Maszk, P., & Losoya, S. (1997). The relations of regulation and emotionality to resiliency and competent social functioning in elementary school children. *Child Development, 68,* 295–311.

Eisenberg, N., & Miller, P. A. (1987). The relation of empathy to prosocial and related behaviors. *Psychological Bulletin, 101,* 91–119.

Eisenberg, N., & Mussen, P. H. (1989). *The roots of prosocial behavior in children.* Cambridge, UK: Cambridge University Press.

Eisenberger, R., & Adornetto, M. (1986). Generalized self-control of delay and effort. *Journal of Personality and Social Psychology, 51,* 1020–1031.

Eisenberger, R., Weier, F., Masterson, F. A., & Theis, L. Y. (1989). Fixed-ratio schedules increase generalized self-control: Preference for large rewards despite high effort or punishment. *Journal of Experimental Psychology: Animal Behavior Processes, 15,* 383–392.

Emde, R. (1992). Social referencing research: Uncertainty, self, and the search for meaning. In S. Feinman (Ed.), *Social referencing and the social construction of reality.* New York: Plenum.

Emde, R., Biringen, Z., Clyman, R., & Oppenhheim, D. (1991). The moral self of infancy: Affective core and procedural knowledge. *Developmental Review, 11,* 251–270.

Emde, R., & Buchsbaum, H. (1990). "Didn't you hear my mommy?": Autonomy with connectedness in moral self-emergence. In D. Cicchetti & M. Beeghly (Eds.), *The self in transition.* Chicago: University of Chicago Press.

Entwisle, D. R., Alexander, K. L., Cadigan, D., & Pallas, A. (1986). The schooling process in first grade: Two samples a decade apart. *American Educational Research Journal, 23,* 587–613.

Entwisle, D. R., & Hayduk, L. A. (1982). *Early schooling: Cognitive and affective outcomes.* Baltimore: Johns Hopkins University Press.

Erickson, M. F., Korfmacher, J., & Egeland, B. (1992). Attachments past and present: Implications for therapeutic interventions with mother-infant dyads. In *Development and Psychopathology.* New York: Cambridge University Press.

Erikson, E. H. (1953). Identity and the life cycle. *Psychological Issues, 1,* 1–171.

Erikson, E. H. (1959). *Identity and the life cycle: Selected papers.* New York: International Universities Press.

Erikson, E. H. (1963). *Childhood and society.* New York: Norton.

Eron, L. D. (1987). The development of aggressive behavior from the perspective of a developing behaviorism. *American Psychologist, 42,* 435–442.

Eysenck, H. J. (1976). The biology of morality. In R. Lickona (Ed.), *Moral development and behavior: Theory, research and social issues.* New York: Holt, Rinehart and Winston.

Fagot, B. I., & Gauvain, M. (1997). Mother–child problem solving: Continuity through the early childhood years. *Child Development, 33,* 480–488.

Fantz, R. L. (1964). Visual experience in infants: Decreased attention to familiar patterns relative to novel ones. *Science, 146,* 668–670.

Fantz, R. L. (1965). Pattern discrimination and selective attention as determinants of perceptual development from birth. In A. M. Kidd & J. L. Riviere (Eds.), *Perceptual development in children.* New York: International University Press.

Fantz, R. L. (1967). Visual perception and experience in early infancy: A look at the hidden side of behavior development. In H. W. Stevenson & H. L. Rheingold (Eds.), *Early behavior.* New York: Wiley.

Farnham-Diggory, S. (1992). *Cognitive processes in education* (2nd ed.). New York: HarperCollins.

Feldman, E., & Dodge, K. A. (1987). Social information processing and sociometric status, sex, age and situational effects. *Journal of Abnormal Child Psychology, 15,* 211–227.

Fenson, L., Kagan, J., Kearsley, R. B., & Zalazo, P. R. (1976). The developmental progression of manipulative play in the first two years. *Child Development, 47,* 232–236.

Festinger, L. (1957). *A theory of cognitive dissonance.* Palo Alto: Stanford University Press.

Festinger, L. (1964a). The motivating effect of cognitive dissonance. In R. S. C. Harper, C. C. Anderson, C. M. Christensen, & S. M. Hunka (Eds.), *The cognitive processes: Readings.* Englewood Cliffs, NJ: Prentice-Hall.

Festinger, L. (1964b). The psychological effects of insufficient rewards. In R. S. C. Harper, C. C. Anderson, C. M. Christensen, & S. M. Hunka (Eds.), *The cognitive processes: Readings.* Englewood Cliffs, NJ: Prentice-Hall.

Finn, J. D., & Cox, D. (1992). Participation and withdrawal among fourth-grade pupils. *American Educational Research Journal, 29,* 141–162.

Fischer, K. W. (1980). A theory of cognitive development: The control and construction of hierarchies of skills. *Psychological Review, 87,* 477–531.

Fischer, K. W., & Rose, S. P. (1994). Dynamic development of coordination of components in brain and behavior: A framework for theory and research. In G. Dawson & K. W. Fischer (Eds.), *Human behavior and the developing brain.* New York: Guilford Press.

Fiske, D. W., & Maddi, S. R. (1961). *Functions of varied experience.* Homewood, NJ: Dorsey Press.

Flavell, J. H. (1971). Stage-related properties of cognitive development. *Cognitive Psychology, 2,* 421–453.

Flavell, J. H. (1977). *Cognitive development.* Englewood Cliffs, NJ: Prentice-Hall.

Flavell, J. H. (1978). Metacognitive development. In J. M. Scandura & C. Brainerd (Eds.), *Structural/process theories of complex human behavior.* Alphenan der Rijn, Netherlands: Sitjoff & Wordhoff.

Flavell, J. H. (1979). Metacognitive and cognitive monitoring: A new area of cognitive–developmental inquiry. *American Psychologist, 34,* 906–911.

Flavell, J. H. (1986). The development of children's knowledge about the appearance–reality distinction. *American Psychologist, 41,* 418–425.

Flavell, J. H. (1993). Young children's understanding of thinking and consciousness. *Current Directions in Psychological Science, 2,* 40–43.

Flavell, J. H., Friedrichs, A. G., & Hoyt, J. D. (1970). Developmental changes in memorization processes. *Cognitive Psychology, 1,* 324–340.

Flavell, J. H., Green, F. L., & Flavell, E. R. (1995). Young children's knowledge about thinking. *Monographs of the Society for Research in Child Development, 60*(1, Serial No. 243).

Flavell, J. H., Green, F. L., Flavell, E. R., & Grossman, J. B. (1997). The development of children's knowledge about inner speech. *Child Development, 68,* 39–47.

Fox, N. A. (Ed.). (1994). The development of emotion regulation: Biological and behavioral considerations. *Monographs of the Society for Research in Child Development, 59*(2–3, Serial No. 240).

Frank, D. A., Klass, P. E., Earls, F., & Eisenberg, L. (1996, April). Infants and young children in orphanages: One view from pediatrics and child psychiatry. *Pediatrics 97,* 569–578.

Freud, A., (1936). *The ego and the mechanisms of defense.* New York: International Universities Press.

Freud, S. (1920). *General introduction to psychoanalysis.* New York: Washington Square Press.

Freud, S. (1923). *The ego and the id.* London: Hogarth Press.

Freud, S. (1930). *Civilization and its discontents.* London: Hogarth Press.

Freud, S. (1955). Beyond the pleasure principle. In J. Strachey (Ed. and Trans.), *The standard edition of the complete psychological works of Sigmund Freud* (Vol. 18). London: Hogarth Press. (Original work published 1920)

Freud, S. (1965). *New introductory lectures on psychoanalysis.* New York: Norton. (Original work published 1932)

Friedman, S. L., Scholnick, E. K., & Cocking, R. R. (1987). Reflections on reflections: What planning is and how it develops. In S. L. Friedman, E. K. Scholnick, & R. R. Cocking (Eds.), *Blueprints for thinking: The role of planning in cognitive development.* Cambridge, UK: Cambridge University Press.

Friedrich, L. K., & Stein, A. H. (1973). Aggressive and prosocial television programs and the natural behavior of preschool children. *Monographs of the Society for Research in Child Development, 38*(4, Serial No. 151), 1–64.

Friedrich-Cofer, L. K., & Huston, A. C. (1986). Television violence and aggression: The debate continues. *Psychological Bulletin, 100,* 364–371.

Fry, P. S. (1984). Teachers' conceptions of students' intelligence and intelligent functioning: A cross-sectional study of elementary, secondary, and tertiary level teachers. In P. S. Fry (Ed.), *Changing conceptions of intelligence and intellectual functioning: Current theory and research.* New York: North-Holland.

Furman, W., & Masters, J. C. (1980). Peer interactions, sociometric status and resistance to deviation in young children. *Developmental Psychology, 16,* 229–236.

Fuson, K. (1979). The development of self-regulating aspects of speech: A review. In G. Zivin (Ed.), *The development of self-regulation through private speech*. New York: Wiley.

Fuster, J. M. (1989). *The prefrontal cortex*. New York: Raven Press.

Garber, J., Braafladt, N., Zeman, J. (1991). The regulation of sad affect: An information processing perspective. In J. Garber & K. Dodge (Eds.), *The development of emotion regulation and dysregulation*. New York: Cambridge University Press.

Gardner, W., & Rogoff, B. (1990). Children's deliberateness of planning according to task circumstances. *Developmental Psychology, 26,* 480–487.

Garvey, C. (1986). Peer relations and the growth of communication. In E. C. Mueller & C. R. Cooper (Eds.), *Process and outcome in peer relationships*. New York: Academic Press.

Gauvain, M., & Rogoff, B. (1989). Collaborative problem-solving and children's planning skills. *Developmental Psychology, 25,* 139–151.

Gazzaniga, M. S. (1985). *The social brain*. New York: Basic Books.

Gazzaniga, M. S. (1992). *Nature's mind: The biological roots of thinking, emotions, sexuality, language, and intelligence*. New York: Basic Books.

Gelman, S. A. (1998). Research in review: Categories in young children's thinking. *Young Children, 53*(1), 20–26.

Gelman, S. A., & Kalish, C. W. (1993). Categories and causality. In R. Pasnak and M. L. Howe (Eds.), *Emerging themes in cognitive development: Vol. II. Competencies*. New York: Springer-Verlag.

Gelman, S. A., & Spelke, E. (1981). The development of thought about animate and inanimate: Implications for research on social cognition. In J. H. Flavell and L. Ross (Eds.), *Social cognitive development: Frontiers and possible futures*. Cambridge, UK: Cambridge University Press.

Gesell, A. L. (1928). *Infancy and human growth*. Old Tappan, NJ: Macmillan.

Gesell, A. L., & Ames, L. B. (1974). *Infant and child in the culture of today* (rev. ed.). New York: Harper & Row.

Getzels, J. W., & Jackson, P. W. (1963). The teacher's personality and characteristics. In N. E. Gage (Ed.), *Handbook of research on teaching*. Chicago: Rand McNally.

Gibson, E. J. (1969). *Principles of perceptual learning and development*. New York: Appleton-Century-Crofts.

Glass, D. C., Reim, B., & Singer, J. E. (1971). Behavioral consequences of adaptation to controllable and uncontrollable noise. *Journal of Experimental Social Psychology, 7,* 244–257.

Goldman-Rakic, P. S. (1987). Circuitry of primate prefrontal cortex and regulation of behavior by representational memory. In F. Plum & V.

Mountcastle (Eds.), *Handbook of physiology: The nervous system* (Vol. 5). Bethesda, MD: American Physiological Society.

Goldman-Rakic, P. S. (1992). Working memory and the mind. *Scientific American, 267,* 110–117.

Goldman-Rakic, P. S. (1993). Specification of higher cortical functions. *Journal of Head Trauma Rehabilitation, 8,* 13–23.

Goldman-Rakic, P. S. (1995). Architecture of the prefrontal cortex and the central executive. In J. Grafman, K. J. Holyoak, & F. Boller (Eds.), *Structure and functions of the human prefrontal cortex: Vol. 769. Annals of the New York Academy of Sciences.* New York: New York Academy of Sciences.

Goodenow, J. (1993). The role of belongingness in adolescents' academic motivation. *Journal of Early Adolescence, 13,* 21–43.

Goodson, B. D. (1982). The development of hierarchic organization: The reproduction, planning, and perception of multi-arch block structures. In G. E. Forman (Ed.), *Action and thought.* New York: Academic Press.

Goodwin, S. H. (1981). The integration of verbal and motor behavior in preschool children. *Child Development, 52,* 280–289.

Graham, S., Harris, K. R., & Reid, R. (1992). Developing self-regulated learners. *Focus on Exceptional Children, 24(6),* 1–16.

Greenfield, P. M. (1971). Goal as environmental variable in the development of intelligence. In R. Cancro (Ed.), *Intelligence: Genetic and environmental influences.* New York: Grune & Stratton.

Greenspan, S. I., & Benderly, B. L. (1997). *The growth of mind and the endangered origins of intelligence.* Reading, MA: Addison Wesley.

Greenwald, A. G. (1980). The totalitarian ego: Fabrication and revision of personal history. *American Psychologist, 35,* 603–618.

Grusec, J. E., & Lytton, H. (1988). *Social development.* New York: Springer-Verlag.

Gulya, M., & Rovee-Collier, C., Galluccio, C., & Wilk, A. (1998). Memory processing of a serial list by young infants. *Psychological Science, 9,* 303–310.

Gunnar, M. R. (1996). *Quality of care and the buffering of stress physiology: Its potential in protecting the developing human brain.* Minneapolis: University of Minnesota Institute of Child Development.

Guralnick, M. J. (1981). Peer influence on the development of communicative competence. In P. Strain (Ed.), *The utilization of classroom peers as behavior change agents.* New York: Plenum.

Hall, C. S. (1954). *A primer of Freudian psychology.* New York: World.

Hardy, D. F., Power, T. G., & Jaedicke, S. (1993). Examining the relation of parenting to children's coping with everyday stress. *Child Development, 64,* 1829–1841.

Harter, S. (1978). Effectance motivation reconsidered: Toward a developmental model. *Human Development, 21,* 34–64.

Harter, S. (1981). A model of mastery motivation in children: Individual differences and developmental change. In W. A. Collins (Ed.), *Aspects on the development of competence: The Minnesota Symposia on Child Psychology* (Vol. 14). Hillsdale, NJ: Erlbaum.

Harter, S. (1983). Developmental perspectives on the self-system. In E. M. Hetherington (Eds.), *Carmichael's manual of child psychology* (4th ed., Vol. 4). New York: Wiley.

Harter, S. (1992). The relationship between perceived competence, affect, and motivational orientation within the classroom: Process and patterns of change. In A. Boggiano & T. Pittman (Eds.), *Achievement and motivation: A social–developmental perspective.* New York: Cambridge University Press.

Harris, K. R. (1982). Cognitive behavior modification: Applications with exceptional students. *Focus on Exceptional Children, 15,* 1–15.

Harris, K. R. (1990). Developing self-regulated learners: The role of private speech and self-instructions. *Educational Psychology, 25,* 35–50.

Harris, K. R., & Graham, S. (1992). Self-regulated strategy development: A part of the writing process. In M. Pressley, K. R. Harris, & J. Guthrie (Eds.), *Promoting academic competence and literacy: Cognitive research and instructional innovation.* New York: Academic Press.

Hartmann, H. (1958). *Ego psychology and the problem of adaptation.* New York: International Universities Press.

Hartup, W. W. (1983). Peer relations. In M. Heatherington (Ed.), *Handbook of child psychology* (Vol. IV). New York: Wiley.

Haste, H. (1987). Growing into rules. In J. Bruner & H. Haste (Eds.), *Making sense: The child's construction of the world.* London: Methuen.

Hauser-Cram, P. (1998). I think I can, I think I can: Understanding and encouraging mastery motivation in young children. *Young Children, 53,* 67–71.

Hauser-Cram, P., Pierson, D., Walker, D. K., & Tivnan, T. (1991). *Early education in the public schools: Lessons from a comprehensive birth-to-kindergarten program.* San Francisco: Jossey-Bass.

Hay, D. F. (1994). Prosocial development. *Journal of Child Psychology and Psychiatry, 35,* 29–72.

Hebb, D. O. (1945). Man's frontal lobes: A critical review. *Archives of Neurology and Psychiatry, 54,* 10–24.

Heckhausen, H. (1968). Achievement motive research: Current problems and some contributions toward a general theory of motivation. In W. J. Arnold (Ed.), *Nebraska Symposium on Motivation.* Lincoln: University of Nebraska Press.

Heider, F. (1958). *The psychology of interpersonal relations.* New York: Wiley.

Helson, H. (1964). *Adaption-level theory.* New York: Harper & Row.

Hendrick, I. (1942). Instinct and the ego during infancy. *Psychoanalytic Quarterly, 11,* 33–58.

Hertz-Lazarowitz, R., & Sharan, S. (1984). Enhancing prosocial behavior through cooperative learning in the classroom. In E. Staub, D. Bar-Tal, J. Karylowski, & J. Reykowski (Eds.), *The development and maintenance of prosocial behavior: International perspectives on positive morality.* New York: Plenum.

Hiroto, D. S. (1974). Locus of control and learned helplessness. *Journal of Experimental Psychology, 102,* 187–193.

Hiroto, D. S., & Seligman, M. E. P. (1975). Generality of learned helplessness in man. *Journal of Personality and Social Psychology, 31,* 311–327.

Hofer, M. A. (1988). On the nature of prenatal behavior. In W. Smotherman & S. Robinson (Eds.), *Behavior of the fetus.* Caldwell, NJ: Telford Press.

Hofer, M. A. (1995). Hidden regulators: Implications for a new understanding of attachment, separation, and loss. In S. Goldberg, R. Muir, & J. Kerr (Eds.), *Attachment theory: social developmental and clinical perspectives.* Hillsdale, NJ: Analytic Press.

Hoffman, M. L. (1970a). Moral development. In P. H. Mussen (Ed.), *Carmichael's manual of child psychology* (3rd ed., Vol. 2). New York: John Wiley & Sons.

Hoffman, M. L. (1970b). Conscience, personality, and socialization techniques. *Human Development, 13,* 90–126.

Hoffman, M. L. (1982). Development of prosocial motivation: Empathy and guilt. In N. Eisenberg (Ed.), *Development of prosocial behavior.* New York: Academic Press.

Hoffman, M. L. (1983). Affective and cognitive processes in moral internalization. In E. T. Higgins, D. N. Ridale, & W. W. Hartup (Eds.), *Social cognition and social development: A sociocultural perspective.* Cambridge, UK: Cambridge University Press.

Hoffman, M. L. (1984). Interaction of affect and cognition in empathy. In C. E. Izard, J. Kagan, & R. Zajonc (Eds.), *Emotions, cognitions, and behavior.* Cambridge, UK: Cambridge University Press.

Hoffman, M. L. (1985). Affect, cognition, and motivation. In R. M. Sorrentino & E. T. Higgins (Eds.), *Handbook of motivation and cognition: Foundations of social behavior* (Vol. 1). New York: Guilford Press.

Hoffman, M. L. (1987). The contributions of empathy to justice and moral judgement. In N. Eisenberg & J. Strayer (Eds.), *Empathy and its development*. Cambridge, UK: Cambridge University Press.

Hofstadter, M., & Resnick, J. S. (1996). Response modality affects human infant delayed-response performance. *Child Development, 67,* 646–658.

Holtz, B. A., & Lehman, E. B. (1995). Development of children's knowledge and use of strategies for self-control in a resistance-to-distraction task. *Merrill-Palmer Quarterly, 41,* 361–380.

Horney, K. (1945). *Our inner conflicts.* New York: Norton.

Howes, C. (1988). Peer interaction of young children. *Monographs of the Society for Research in Child Development, 53*(1, Serial No. 217), 1–88.

Howes, C. (1990). Social status and friendship from kindergarten to third grade. *Journal of Applied Developmental Psychology, 11,* 321–330.

Hudson, J. A., & Fivush, R. (1991). Planning in the preschool years: The emergence of plans from general event knowledge. *Cognitive Development, 6,* 393–415.

Hughes, J. N. (1988). *Cognitive behavior therapy with children in schools.* New York: Pergamon.

Hull, C. L. (1943). *Principles of behavior: An introduction to behavior theory.* New York: Appleton-Century-Crofts.

Hull, C. L. (1952). *A behavior system: An introduction to behavior theory concerning the individual organism.* New Haven, CT: Yale University Press.

Hunt, J. M. (1960). Experience and the development of motivation: Some reinterpretations. *Child Development, 31,* 489–504.

Hunt, J. M. (1961). *Intelligence and experience.* New York: Ronald Press.

Hunt, J. M. (1963). Motivation inherent in information processing and action. In O. J. Harvey (Ed.), *Motivation and social interaction: Cognitive determinants.* New York: Ronald Press.

Hunt, J. M. (1965). Intrinsic motivation and its role in psychological development. In D. Levine (Ed.), *Nebraska Symposium on Motivation.* Lincoln: University of Nebraska Press.

Hunt, J. M. (1966). The epigenesis of intrinsic motivation and early cognitive learning. In R. N. Haber (Ed.), *Current research in motivation.* New York: Holt, Rinehart and Winston.

Huttenlocher, P. R. (1993). Morphometric study of human cerebral cortex development. In M. H. Johnson (Ed.), *Brain development and cognition: A reader.* Oxford, UK: Blackwell.

Iannotti, R. J. (1978). Effect of role-taking experiences on role-taking, empathy, altruism, and aggression. *Developmental Psychology, 14,* 119–124.

Inhelder, B., & Piaget, J. (1964). *The early growth of logic in the child.* New York: Norton.

Jensen, E. (1998). *Teaching with the brain in mind.* Alexandria, VA: Association for Supervision and Curriculum Development.

Jennings, K. D. (1993). Mastery motivation and the formation of self-concept from infancy through early childhood. In D. J. Messer (Ed.), *Mastery motivation in early childhood: Development, measurement and social processes.* London: Routledge.

Johnson, C. N., & Wellman, H. M. (1982). Children's developing conceptions of mind and brain. *Child Development, 53,* 222–234.

Johnson, D. (1991). *Learning together and alone: Cooperative, competitive, and individualistic learning.* Englewood Cliffs, NJ: Prentice-Hall.

Johnson, D., Johnson, R., Johnson-Holubee, E., & Roy, P. (1984). *Circles of learning: Cooperation in the classroom.* Alexandria, VA: Association for Supervision and Curriculum Development.

Kagan, J. (1958). The concept of identification. *Psychological Review, 65,* 296–305.

Kagan, J. (1971). *Change and continuity in infancy.* New York: Wiley.

Kagan, J. (1997). Temperament and the reactions to unfamiliarity. *Child Development, 68,* 139–147.

Kail, R. (1990). *The development of memory in children* (3rd ed.). New York: Freeman.

Kandel, D. B., & Lesser, G. S. (1972). *Youth in two worlds.* San Francisco: Jossey-Bass.

Karmiloff-Smith, A. (1979). *A functional approach to child language.* Cambridge, UK: Cambridge University Press.

Karmiloff-Smith, A. (1986). Stage/structure versus phase/process in modeling linguistic and cognitive development. In I. Levin (Ed.), *Stage and structure: Reopening the debate.* Norwood, NJ: Ablex.

Karmiloff-Smith, A. (1993). Self-organization and cognitive change. In M. H. Johnson (Ed.), *Brain development and cognition.* Oxford, UK: Blackwell.

Karmiloff-Smith, A. (1995). Annotation: The extraordinary cognitive journey from foetus through infancy. *Journal of Child Psychology and Psychiatry and Allied Disciplines, 36,* 1293–1313.

Katz, L. G., & McClellan, D. E. (1997). *Fostering children's social competence: The teacher's role.* Washington, DC: National Association for the Education of Young Children.

Kelley, H. H. (1967). Attribution theory in social psychology. In D. Levine (Ed.), *Nebraska Symposium on Motivation* (Vol. 15). Lincoln: University of Nebraska Press.

Kemple, K. (1991). Preschool children's peer acceptance and social interaction. *Young Children, 46,* 47–54.

Kirby, J. R. (1984). Educational roles of cognitive plans and strategies. In J. R. Kirby (Ed.), *Cognitive strategies and educational performance.* New York: Academic Press.

Kirby, J. R., & Ashman, A. F. (1984). Planning skills and mathematics achievement. *Journal of Psychoeducational Assessment, 2,* 9-22.

Klahr, D., & Robinson, M. (1981). Formal assessment of problem-solving and planning processes in preschool children. *Cognitive Psychology, 13,* 113–148.

Klinnert, M. D., Campos, J. J., Sorce, J. F., Emde, R. N., & Svejda, M. (1983). Emotions as behavior regulators: Social referencing in infancy. In R. Plutchik and H. Kellerman (Eds.), *Emotion: Theory, research, and experience* (Vol. 2). New York: Academic Press.

Kochanska, G. (1991). Socialization and temperament in the development of guilt and conscience. *Child Development, 62,* 1379–1392.

Kochanska, G. (1993). Toward a synthesis of parental socialization and child temperament in early development of conscience. *Child Development, 64,* 325–347.

Koffka, K. (1935). *Principles of Gestalt psychology.* New York: Harcourt, Brace.

Kohlberg, L. (1969). Stage and sequence: The cognitive–developmental approach to socialization. In D. A. Goslin (Ed.), *Handbook of socialization theory and research.* Chicago: Rand McNally.

Kohler, W. (1947). *Gestalt psychology: An introduction to new concepts in modern psychology.* New York: Liveright.

Kohler, W. (1959). Gestalt psychology today. *American Psychologist, 14,* 727–734.

Kohler, W. (1969). *The task of Gestalt psychology.* Princeton, NJ: Princeton University Press.

Kopp, C. B. (1982). Antecedents of self-regulation: A developmental perspective. *Developmental Psychology, 18,* 199–214.

Kopp, C. B. (1989). Regulation of distress and negative emotions: A developmental view. *Developmental Psychology, 25,* 343–354.

Kopp, C. B. (1992). Emotional distress and control in young children. In N. Eisenberg & R. A. Fabes (Eds.), *Emotion and its regulation in early development: New directions for child development.* San Francisco: Jossey-Bass.

Krebs, D., & Sturrup, B. (1982). Role-taking ability and altruistic behavior in elementary school children. *Journal of Moral Education, 11,* 94–100.

Kreitler, S., & Kreitler, H. (1987). Conceptions and processes of planning. In S. L. Friedman, E. K. Scholnick, & R. R. Cocking (Eds.), *Blueprints for thinking: The role of planning in cognitive development.* Cambridge, UK: Cambridge University Press.

Kuczynski, L., & Kochanska, G. (1995). Function and content of maternal demands: Developmental significance of early demands for competent action. *Child Development, 66,* 616–628.

Kuhn, D., & Phelps, E. (1982). The development of problem-solving strategies. In H. Reese (Ed.), *Advances in child development and behavior* (Vol. 17). New York: Academic Press.

Kupersmidt, J. B., Coie, J. D., & Dodge, K. A. (1990). The role of poor peer relationships in the development of disorder. In S. R. Asher & J. D. Coie (Eds.), *Peer rejection in childhood.* New York: Cambridge University Press.

Ladd, G. W., & Price, J. M. (1989). Predicting children's social and school adjustment following the transition from preschool to kindergarten. *Child Development, 58,* 1168–1189.

Ladd, G. W., Price, J. M., & Hart, C. H. (1990). Preschoolers' behavioral orientations and patterns of peer contact: Predictive of peer status. In S. Asher & J. Coie (Eds.), *Peer rejection in childhood.* New York: Cambridge University Press.

Larsen, R. J., Diener, E., & Cropanzano, R. A. (1987). Cognitive operations associated with individual differences in affect intensity, *Journal of Personality and Social Psychology, 53,* 767-774.

Lazar, I., & Darlington, R. (1982). Lasting effects of early education: A report from the Consortium for Longitudinal Studies. *Monograph of the Society for Research in Child Development, 47*(2–3, Serial No. 195).

Lazarus, R. (1966). *Psychological stress and the coping process.* New York: McGraw-Hill.

LeDoux, J. (1996). *The emotional brain.* New York: Simon & Schuster.

Lepper, M. R. (1981). Intrinsic and extrinsic motivation in children: Detrimental effects of superfluous social controls. In W. A. Collins (Ed.), *Minnesota Symposium on Child Psychology* (Vol. 14). Minneapolis: University of Minnesota Press.

Lepper, M. R. (1983). Social-control processes and the internalization of social values: An attributional perspective. In E. T. Higgins, D. N. Rible, & W. W. Hartup (Eds.), *Social cognition and social development: A sociocultural perspective.* Cambridge, UK: Cambridge University Press.

Lepper, M. R., & Greene, D. (1978). Overjustification research and beyond: Toward a means-ends analysis of intrinsic and extrinsic motivation. In M. R. Lepper & D. Greene (Eds.), *The hidden costs of reward: New perspectives on the psychology of human motivation.* Hillsdale, NJ: Erlbaum.

Lepper, M. R., & Hodell, M. (1989). Intrinsic motivation in the classroom. In C. Ames & R. Ames (Eds.), *Research on motivation in education* (Vol. 3). San Diego: Academic Press.

Lewis, M., & Brooks-Gunn, J. (1979). *Social cognition and the acquisition of self.* New York: Plenum.

Lezak, M. D. (1982). The problem of assessing executive functions. *International Journal of Psychology, 17,* 281–297.

Lezak, M. D. (1983). *Neuropsychological assessment* (2nd ed.). New York: Oxford University Press.

Light, P. (1987). Taking roles. In J. Bruner & H. Haste (Eds.), *Making sense.* London: Methuen.

Loftus, E. F., & Palmer, J. C. (1974). Reconstruction of automobile destruction: An example of the interaction between language and memory. *Journal of Verbal Learning and Verbal Behavior, 13,* 585–589.

Logue, A. W. (1995). *Self-control.* Englewood Cliffs, NJ: Prentice-Hall.

Londerville, S., & Main, M. (1981). Security of attachment, compliance, and maternal training methods in the second year of life. *Developmental Psychology, 17,* 298–299.

Lorenz, K. (1965). *Evolution and modification of behavior.* Chicago: University of Chicago Press.

Lorenz, K. (1966). *On aggression.* London: Methuen.

Luria, A. R. (1961). *The role of speech in the regulation of normal and abnormal behavior.* London: Pergamon.

Luria, A. R. (1972). *The working brain.* Harmondsworth, UK: Penguin.

Luria, A. R. (1976). *Cognitive development: Its cultural and social foundations.* Cambridge, MA: Harvard University Press.

Luria, A. R. (1980). *Higher cortical functions in man* (2nd ed.). New York: Basic Books.

Maccoby, E. E. (1980). *Social development: Psychological growth and the parent–child relationship.* San Diego: Harcourt, Brace, Jovanovich.

Maier, S. F., & Seligman, M. E. P. (1976). Learned helplessness: Theory and evidence. *Journal of Experimental Psychology: General, 105,* 3–46.

Mandler, G. (1975). *Mind and emotion.* New York: Wiley.

Manly, T., & Robertson, I. H. (1997). Sustained attention and the frontal lobes. In P. Rabbitt (Ed.), *Methodology of frontal and executive function.* East Sussex, UK: Psychology Press.

Maratsos, M. P. (1983). Some current issues in the study of the acquisition of grammar. In J. H. Flavell & E. Markman (Eds.), *Handbook of child psychology* (Vol. 3). New York: Wiley.

Markman, E. M. (1979). Realizing that you don't understand: Elementary school children's awareness of inconsistencies. *Child Development, 50,* 643–655.

Markus, H. (1977). Self-schemas and processing information about the self. *Journal of Personality and Social Psychology, 35,* 63–78.

Markus, H., & Nurius, P. (1986). Possible selves. *American Psychologist, 41,* 954–969.

Maslow, A. H. (1968). *Toward a psychology of being* (2nd ed.). New York: Van Nostrand.

Maslow, A. H. (1970). *Motivation and personality* (2nd ed.). New York: Harper & Row.

Masters, J. C., & Binger, C. G. (1978). Interrupting the flow of behavior: The stability and development of children's initiation and maintenance of compliant response inhibition. *Merrill Palmer Quarterly, 24,* 229–242.

May, R. (1953). *Man's search for himself.* New York: Norton.

May, R. (1967). *Psychology and the human dilemma.* New York: Van Nostrand.

May, R. (1969). *Love and will.* New York: Norton.

McCall, R. B., & Kagan, J. (1970). Individual differences in the infant's distribution of attention to stimulus discrepancy. *Developmental Psychology, 2,* 90–98.

McClelland, D. C. (1966). Importance of early learning in the formation of motives. In R. N. Haber (Ed.), *Current research in motivation.* New York: Holt Rinehart and Winston.

McClelland, D. C., Atkinson, J. W., Clark, R. W., & Lowell, E. L. (1953). *The achievement motive.* New York: Appleton-Century-Crofts.

McGillicuddy-DeLisi, A. V., DeLisi, R., Flaugher, J., & Sigel, I. E. (1987). Familial influences on planning. In S. L. Friedman, E. K. Scholnick, & R. R. Cocking (Eds.), *Blueprints for thinking: The role of planning in cognitive development.* Cambridge, UK: Cambridge University Press.

McKim, B., & Cowen, E. L. (1987). Multiperspective assessment of young children's school adjustment. *School Psychology Review, 16,* 370–381.

Meichenbaum, D. (1977). *Cognitive behavior modification: An integrative approach.* New York: Plenum.

Meichenbaum, D. (1984). Teaching thinking: A cognitive behavioral perspective. In J. Sigal, S. Chipman, & R. Glaser (Eds.), *Thinking and learning skills* (Vol. 2). Hillsdale, NJ: Erlbaum.

Meichenbaum, D., & Asernow, J. (1979). Cognitive behavior modification and metacognitive development: Implications for the classroom. In P. C. Kendall & D. Hollon (Eds.), *Cognitive behavioral interventions: Theory, research, and procedures.* New York: Academic Press.

Meltzoff, A. N. (1995). Understanding the intentions of others: Re-enactment of intended acts by 18-month-old children. *Developmental Psychology, 31,* 838–850.

Miller, G. A., Galanter, E., & Pribram, K. H. (1960). *Plans and the structure of behavior.* New York: Holt, Rinehart and Winston.

Miller, N. A., & Dollard, J. C. (1941). *Social learning and imitation.* New Haven, CT: Yale University Press.

Minuchin, P. (1971). Correlates of curiosity and exploratory behavior in preschool disadvantaged children. *Child Development, 42,* 939–950.

Mischel, H. N., & Mischel, W. (1983). Development of children's knowledge of self-control strategies. *Child Development, 54,* 603–619.

Mischel, W. (1974). Processes in delay of gratification. In L. Berkowitz (Ed.), *Advances in experimental social psychology* (Vol. 7). New York: Academic Press.

Mischel, W., & Patterson, C. J. (1979). Effective plans for self-control in children. In A. Collins (Ed.), *Minnesota Symposium on Child Psychology.* Hillsdale, NJ: Erlbaum.

Mischel, W., Shoda, Y., & Rodriguez, M. L. (1989). Delay of gratification in children. *Science, 244,* 933–938.

Miserandino, M. (1996). Children who do well in school: Individual differences in perceived competence and autonomy in above average children. *Journal of Educational Psychology, 88,* 203–214.

Mize, J., & Ladd, G. (1990). Toward the development of successful social skills training for preschool children. In S. R. Asher & J. D. Coie (Eds.), *Peer rejection in childhood.* New York: Cambridge University Press.

Mlot, C. (1998). Probing the biology of emotion. *Science, 280,* 1005–1007.

Morgan, G. A., Harmon, R. J., & Maslin-Cole, C. A. (1990). Mastery motivation: Definition and measurement. *Early Education and Development, 1,* 318–339.

Morgan, G. A., Maslin-Cole, C. A., Biringer, Z., & Harmon, R. J. (1991). Play assessment of mastery motivation in infants and young children. In C. E. Schaefer, K. Gitlin, & A. Sandgrund (Eds.), *Play diagnosis and assessment.* New York: Wiley.

Mumme, D. L., Fernald, A., & Herrera, C. (1996). Infants' responses to facial and vocal emotional signals in a social referencing paradigm. *Child Development, 67,* 3219–3237.

Naglieri, J. A., & Das, J. P. (1987). Construct and criterion related validity of planning, simultaneous and successive cognitive processing tasks. *Journal of Psychoeducational Assessment, 4,* 353–363.

Nelson, K. (1979). The role of language in infant development. In M. Bornstein & W. Kessen (Eds.), *Psychological development from infancy: Image to intention.* Hillsdale, NJ: Erlbaum.

Nelson, K. (Ed.). (1986). *Event knowledge: Structure and function in development*. Hillsdale, NJ: Erlbaum.

Nelson-Le Gall, S. (1992). Children's instrumental help seeking: Its role in the social acquisition and skill. In R. Hertz-Lazarowitz & N. Miller (Eds.), *Interaction in cooperative groups: The theoretical anatomy of group learning*. New York: Cambridge University Press.

Norman, D. A., & Shallice, T. (1986). Attention to action: Willed and automatic control of behavior. In R. J. Davidson, G. E. Schwartz, & D. Shapiro (Eds.), *Consciousness and self-regulation: Advances in research* (Vol. 4). New York: Plenum.

Nucci, L. P., Killen, M., & Smetana, J. G. (1996). Autonomy and the personal: Negotiation and social reciprocity in adult–child social exchanges. In M. Killen (Ed.), *New directions for child development: No. 73. Children's autonomy, social competence, and interactions with adults and other children: Exploring connections and consequences*. San Francisco: Jossey-Bass.

Odom, S. L., McConnell, S. R., & McEvoy, M. A. (1992). Peer related social competence and its significance for young children with disabilities. In S. L. Odom, S. R. McConnell, & M. A. McEvoy (Eds.), *Social competence of young children with disabilities*. Baltimore: Brooks.

O'Leary, S., & Dubey, D. (1979). Applications of self-control procedures by children: A review. *Journal of Applied Behavior Analysis, 12,* 449–465.

Oliner, S. P., & Oliner, P. M. (1988). *The altruistic personality: Rescuers of Jews in Nazi Europe*. New York: Free Press.

Palincsar, A. S., & Brown, A. L. (1984). Reciprocal teaching of comprehension-fostering and comprehension-monitoring activities. *Cognition and Instruction, 1,* 117–175.

Pallas, A. M., Entwisle, D. R., Alexander, K. C., & Cadigan, D. (1987). Children who do exceptionally well in first grade. *Sociology of Education, 60,* 256–271.

Papousek, H. (1967). Experimental studies of appetitional behavior in human newborns and infants. In H. W. Stevenson, E. H. Hess, & H. L. Rheingold (Eds.), *Early behavior*. New York: Wiley.

Papousek, H. (1969). Individual variability in learning responses in human infants. In R. J. Robinson (Ed.), *Brain and early behavior*. London: Academic Press.

Paris, S. G., & Ayres, L. R. (1994). *Becoming reflective students and teachers: With portfolios and authentic assessment*. Washington, DC: American Psychological Association.

Paris, S. G, & Byrnes, J. P. (1989). The constructivist approach to self-regulation and learning in the classroom. In B. J. Zimmerman & D. H.

Schunk (Eds.), *Self-regulated learning and academic achievement: Theory, research, and practice*. New York: Springer-Verlag.

Paris, S. G., & Lindauer, B. K. (1982). The development of cognitive skills during childhood. In B. Wolman (Ed.), *Handbook of developmental psychology*. Englewood Cliffs, NJ: Prentice-Hall.

Parke, R. D., & Slaby, R. G. (1983). The development of aggression. In E. M. Hetherington (Ed.), *Handbook of child psychology* (4th ed., Vol. 4). New York: Wiley.

Parker, J. G., & Asher, S. R. (1987). Peer relations and later personal adjustment: Are low accepted children at risk? *Psychological Bulletin, 102,* 357–389.

Parker, J. G., & Gottman, J. M. (1989). Social and emotional development in a relational context: Friendship interactions from early childhood to adolescence. In T. Berndt & G. Ladd (Eds.), *Peer relationships in child development*. New York: Wiley.

Parten, M. (1932). Social participation among preschool children. *Journal of Abnormal and Social Psychology, 27,* 243–269.

Pasnak, R., & Howe, M. L. (1993). New approaches to the development of cognitive competence. In R. Pasnak & M. L. Howe (Eds.), *Emerging themes in cognitive development: Vol. II. Competencies*. New York: Springer-Verlag.

Passingham, R. (1993). *Oxford psychology series: No. 21. The frontal lobes and voluntary action*. Oxford, UK: Oxford University Press.

Patterson, G. R. (1986). Maternal rejection: Determinant or product of deviant child behavior? In W. W. Hartup & Z. Rubin (Eds.), *Relationships and development*. Hillsdale, NJ: Erlbaum.

Pavlov, I. P. (1927). *Conditioned reflexes*. London: Oxford University Press.

Pellegrini, A. D. (1992). Kindergarten children's social cognitive status as a predictor of first-grade success. *Early Childhood Research Quarterly, 7,* 565–577.

Perry, B. D. (1996). Incubated in terror: Neurodevelopmental factors in the "cycle of violence." In J. D. Osovsky (Ed.), *Children in a violent society*. New York: Guilford Press.

Phares, E. J. (1976). *Locus of control in personality*. Morristown, NJ: General Learning Press.

Piaget, J. (1926). *Language and thought of the child*. London: Routledge & Kegan Paul.

Piaget, J. (1950). *The psychology of intelligence*. London: Routledge & Kegan Paul.

Piaget, J. (1952). *The origins of intelligence in children*. New York: International Universities Press.

Piaget, J. (1954). *The construction of reality in the child.* New York: Basic Books.

Piaget, J. (1962). *Play, dreams, and imitation in childhood.* New York: Norton.

Piaget, J. (1965). *The moral judgment of the child.* New York: Free Press.

Piaget, J. (1967). *Six psychological studies.* New York: Random House.

Piaget, J. (1970). Piaget's theory. In P. H. Mussen (Ed.), *Carmichael's manual of child psychology* (3rd ed., Vol. 1). New York: Wiley.

Piaget, J. (1973). *To understand is to invent: The future of education.* New York: Grossman.

Piaget, J. (1985). *The equilibration of cognitive structures: The central problem of intellectual development.* Chicago: University of Chicago Press.

Piaget, J., & Inhelder, B. (1969). *The psychology of the child.* New York: Basic Books.

Pintrich, P. R., & DeGroot, E. V. (1990). Motivational and self-regulated learning components of classroom academic performance. *Journal of Educational Psychology, 82,* 33–40.

Pintrich, P. R., & Schunk, D. H. (1996). *Motivation in education: Theory, research and applications.* Englewood Cliffs, NJ: Prentice-Hall.

Posner, M. I., & Presti, D. F. (1987). Selective attention and cognitive control. *Trends in Neuroscience, 10,* 13.

Prawat, R. S. (1998). Current self-regulation views of learning and motivation viewed through a Deweyan lens: The problems with dualism. *American Educational Research Journal, 35,* 199–224.

Pressley, M. Harris, K. R., & Marks, M. B. (1992). But good strategy instructors are constructivists! *Educational Psychology Review, 4,* 3–31.

Pressley, M., Woloshyn, V., Lysynchuk, L. M., Martin, V., Wood, E., & Willoughby, T. (1990). A primer of research on cognitive strategy instruction: The important issues and how to address them. *Educational Psychology Review, 2,* 1–58.

Prevost, R. A., Bronson, M. B., & Casey, M. B. (1995). Planning processes in preschool children. *Journal of Applied Developmental Psychology, 16,* 505–527.

Putallaz, M. (1983). Predicting children's sociometric status from their behavior. *Child Development, 54,* 1417–1426.

Putallaz, M., & Gottman, J. M. (1981). An interactional model of children's entry into peer groups. *Child Development, 52,* 986–994.

Quinn, P. C., Eimas, P. D., & Rosenkrantz, S. L. (1993). Evidence for representations of perceptually similar natural categories by 3-month-old and 4-month-old infants. *Perception, 22,* 463–475.

Rabbit, P. (1997). *Methodology of frontal and executive function.* East Sussex, UK: Psychology Press.

Redding, R. E., Morgan, G. A., & Harmon, R. J. (1988). Mastery motivation in infants and toddlers: Is it greatest when tasks are moderately challenging? *Infant Behavior and Development, 11,* 419–430.

Renken, B., Egeland, B., Marvinney, D., Mangelsdorf, S., & Sroufe, L. A. (1989). Early childhood antecedents of aggression and passive-withdrawal in early elementary school. *Journal of Personality, 57,* 257–281.

Reynolds, A. J. (1991). Early schooling of children at risk. *American Educational Research Journal, 28,* 392–422.

Rheingold, H. L. (1982). Little children's participation in the work of adults, a nascent prosocial behavior. *Child Development, 53,* 114–125.

Rheingold, H. L., Hay, D. F., & West, M. J. (1976). Sharing the second year of life. *Child Development, 47,* 118–1158.

Robinson, J. L., Zahn-Waxler, C., & Emde, R. (1994). Patterns of development in early empathetic behavior: Environmental and child contributional influences. *Social Development, 3,* 125–145.

Rodriguez, M. L., Mischel, W., & Shoda, Y. (1989). Cognitive person variables in the delay of gratification of older children at risk. *Journal of Personality and Social Psychology, 57,* 358–367.

Rogers, C. R. (1963). Actualizing endency in relation to motives and to consciousness. In M. R. Jones (Ed.), *Nebraska Symposium on Motivation.* Lincoln: University of Nebraska Press.

Rogoff, B. (1986). The development of strategic use of context in spatial memory. In M. Perlmutter (Ed.), *Perspectives on intellectual development.* Hillsdale, NJ: Erlbaum.

Rogoff, B. (1990). *Apprenticeship in thinking: Cognitive development in social context.* New York: Oxford University Press.

Rogoff, B., & Gardner, W. P. (1984). Guidance in cognitive development: An examination of mother–child instruction. In B. Rogoff & J. Lave (Eds.), *Everyday cognition: Its development in social context.* Cambridge, MA: Harvard University Press.

Rose-Krasnor, L., Rubin, K. H., Booth, C. L., & Coplan, R. (1996). The relation of maternal directiveness and child attachment security to social competence in preschoolers. *International Journal of Behavioral Development, 19,* 309–325.

Rothbart, M. K., Ziaie, H., & O'Boyle, C. G. (1992). Self-regulation and emotion in infancy. In N. Eisenberg & R. A. Fabes (Eds.), *New directions for child development: No. 55. Emotion and its regulation in early development.* San Francisco: Jossey-Bass.

Rothbaum, F., & Crockenberg, S. (1995). Maternal control and two-year-olds' compliance and defiance. *International Journal of Behavioral Development, 18,* 193–210.

Rotter, J. B. (1966). Generalized expectancies for internal versus external control of reinforcement. *Psychological Monographs, 80*(1, No. 609).

Rotter, J. B., Seaman, M., & Liverant, S. (1962). Internal versus external control of reinforcement: A major variable in behavior theory. In N. F. Washburn (Ed.), *Decisions, values, and groups.* New York: Pergamon.

Rovee-Collier, C. (1989). The joy of kicking: Memories, motives, and mobiles. In P. Soloman, G. Goethals, C. Kelly, & B. Stephens (Eds.), *Memory: Interdisciplinary approaches.* New York: Springer-Verlag.

Rubin, K. H., Chen, X., & Hymel, S. (1993). Socio-emotional characteristics of withdrawn and aggressive children. *Merrill-Palmer Quarterly, 39,* 518–534.

Rubin, K. H., Hymel, S., & Mills, R. S. L. (1989). Sociability and social withdrawals in childhood: Stability and outcomes. *Journal of Personality, 57,* 237–255.

Rubin, K. H., & Pepler, D. J. (1980). The relationship of children's play to social cognitive growth and development. In H. Foot, A. Chapmen, & J. Smith (Eds.), *Friendship and social relations in children.* New York: Wiley.

Rubin, K. H., & Rose-Krasnor, L. (1992). Interpersonal problem solving and social competence in children. In V. B. Van Hasselt & M. Hersen (Eds.), *Handbook of social development: A lifespan perspective.* New York: Plenum.

Rudolph, K. D., Harmen, C., & Burge, D. (1995). Cognitive representations of self, family, and peers in school competence and sociometric status. *Child Development, 66,* 1385–1402.

Rushton, J. P., Fulker, D. W. Neale, M. L., Nias, D. K., & Eysenck, H. J. (1986). Altruism and aggression: The heritability of individual differences. *Journal of Personality and Social Psychology, 50,* 1192–1198.

Russell, A., & Russell, G. (1996). Positive parenting and boys' and girls' misbehavior during a home observation. *International Journal of Behavioral Development, 19,* 291–307.

Rutherford, E., & Mussen, P. H. (1968). Generosity in nursery school boys. *Child Development, 39,* 755–765.

Ryan, R. M. (1993). Agency and organization: Intrinsic motivation, autonomy, and the self in psychological development. In J. E. Jacobs (Ed.), *Nebraska Symposium on Motivation 1992* (Vol. 40). Lincoln: University of Nebraska Press.

Ryan, R. M., & Grolnick, W. S. (1986). Origins and pawns in the classroom: Self-report and projective assessments of individual differences in children's perspectives. *Journal of Personality and Social Psychology, 50,* 550–558.

Ryan, R. M., & Powelson, C. L. (1991). Autonomy and relatedness as fundamental to motivation and education. *Journal of Experimental Education, 60,* 49–66.

Ryan, R. M., & Stiller, J. (1991). The social context of internalization: Parent and teacher influences on autonomy, motivation, and learning. In M. L. Maehr & P. R. Pintrich (Eds.), *Advances in motivation and achievement* (Vol. 7). Greenwich, CT: JAI Press.

Sandler, I. N., Tein, J., & West, S. G. (1994). Coping, stress and the psychological symptoms of children of divorce: A cross-sectional and longitudinal study. *Child Development, 65,* 1744–1763.

Scaife, M., & Bruner, J. S. (1975). The capacity for joint visual attention in the infant. *Nature, 253,* 265–266.

Schachter, S., & Singer, J. E. (1962). Cognitive, social and physiological determinants of emotional state. *Psychological Review, 69,* 379–399.

Schaffer, H. R. (1996). *Social development.* Oxford, UK: Blackwell.

Scholnick, E. K., & Friedman, S. L. (1987). The planning construct in the psychological literature. In S. L. Friedman, E. K. Scholnick, & R. R. Cocking (Eds.),*Blueprints for thinking: The role of planning in cognitive development.* Cambridge, UK: Cambridge University Press.

Schore, A. N. (1994). *Affect regulation and the origin of the self: The neurobiology of emotional development.* Hillsdale, NJ: Erlbaum.

Schunk, D. H. (1989). Self-efficacy and cognitive skill learning. In C. Ames & R. Ames (Eds.), *Research on motivation in education* (Vol. 3). Orlando: Academic Press.

Schunk, D. H. (1991). Self-efficacy and academic motivation. *Educational Psychologist, 26,* 207–231.

Schunk, D. H., & Zimmerman, B. J. (1994). *Self-regulation of learning and performance: Issues and educational applications.* Hillsdale, NJ: Erlbaum.

Schunk, S. Z., Schunk, A., Hallam, E., Mancini, F., & Wells, R. (1971). Sex differences in aggressive behavior subsequent to listening to a radio broadcast of violence. *Psychological Reports, 28,* 931–936.

Schweder, R. A. (1991). *Thinking through cultures: Expeditions in cultural psychology.* Cambridge, MA: Harvard University Press.

Seligman, M. E. P. (1975). *Helplessness.* San Francisco: Freeman.

Seligman, M. E. P. (1991). *Learned optimism.* New York: Knopf.

Seligman, M. E. P., & Maier, S. F. (1967). Failure to escape traumatic shock. *Journal of Experimental Psychology, 74,* 1–9.

Shallice, T. (1988). *From neuropsychology to mental structure.* Cambridge, UK: Cambridge University Press.

Shallice, T., & Burgess, P. (1991). Deficits in strategy application following frontal lobe damage in man. *Brain, 114,* 727–741.

Shapiro, E. S. (1984). Self-monitoring procedures. In T. H. Ollendick & M.

Herson (Eds.), *Child behavior assessment: Principles and procedures.* New York: Pergamon.

Shatz, M., Wellman, H. M., & Silber, S. (1983). The acquisition of mental verbs: A systematic investigation of the first reference to mental state. *Cognition, 14,* 301–322.

Shore, R. (1997). *Rethinking the brain: New insights into early development.* New York: Families and Work Institute.

Shure, M. B. (1981). Social competence as problem-solving skill. In J. Wine & M. Smye (Eds.), *Social competence.* New York: Guilford Press.

Siegler, R. S. (1984). Mechanisms of cognitive growth: Variation and selection. In R. J. Sternberg (Ed.), *Mechanisms of cognitive development.* New York: Freeman.

Siegler, R. S. (1986). Unities in strategy choices across domains. In M. Perlmutter (Ed.), *Minnesota Symposium on Child Development* (Vol. 19). Hillsdale, NJ: Erlbaum.

Siegler, R. S. (1987). Strategy choices in subtraction. In J. Sloboda & D. Rogers (Eds.), *Cognitive process in mathematics.* Oxford, UK: Oxford University Press.

Siegler, R. S. (1988a). Strategy choice procedures and the development of multiplication skill. *Journal of Experimental Psychology: General, 117,* 258–275.

Siegler, R. S. (1988b). Individual differences in strategy choices: Good students, not-so-good students, and perfectionists. *Child Development, 59,* 833–851.

Siegler, R. S. (1989). Mechanisms of cognitive development. *Annual Review of Psychology, 40,* 353–379.

Siegler, R. S., & Jenkins, E. (1989). *How children discover new strategies.* New York: Erlbaum.

Siegman, A. W. (1961). The relationship between future time perspective, time estimation, and impulse control in a group of young offenders and in a control group. *Journal of Consulting Psychology, 25,* 470–475.

Skinner, B. F. (1938). *The behavior of organisms: An experimental analysis.* Englewood Cliffs, NJ: Prentice-Hall.

Skinner, B. F. (1948). *Walden Two.* New York: Macmillan.

Skinner, B. F. (1957). *Verbal behavior.* New York: Appleton-Century-Crofts.

Skinner, B. F. (1974). *About behaviorism.* New York: Knopf.

Skinner, E. A. (1986). The origins of young children's perceived control: Caregiver contingent and sensitive behavior. *International Journal of Behavioral Development, 9,* 359–382.

Skinner, E. A., Zimmer-Gembeck, M. J., & Connell, J. P. (1998). Individual differences and the development of perceived control. *Monographs of the Society for Research in Child Development, 63*(2–3 Serial No. 254).

Solomon, D., Watson, M., Schaps, E., Battistich, V., & Solomon, J. (1990). Cooperative learning as part of a comprehensive program designed to promote prosocial development. In S. Sharan (Ed.), *Current research on cooperative learning.* New York: Praeger.

Spitz, R. A. (1945). Hospitalism: An inquiry into the genesis of psychiatric conditions in early childhood. *Psychoanalytic Study of the Child, 1,* 53–74.

Spivack, G., Platt, J. J., & Shure, M. B. (1976). *The problem-solving approach to adjustment.* San Francisco: Jossey-Bass.

Sroufe, L. A. (1988). The role of infant–caregiver attachment in development. In J. Belsky & T. Nezworski (Eds.), *Clinical implications of attachment.* Hillsdale, NJ: Erlbaum.

Sroufe, L. A. (1989). Infant–caregiver attachment and patterns of adaptation in preschool: The roots of maladaptation and competence. In M. Perlmutter (Ed.), *Minnesota Symposium in Child Psychology* (Vol. 19). Hillsdale, NJ: Erlbaum.

Sroufe, L. A. (1995). *Emotional development: The organization of emotional life in the early years.* Cambridge, UK: Cambridge University Press.

Sroufe, L. A., Carlson, E., & Schulman, S. (1993). Individuals in relationships: Development from infancy through adolescence. In D. C. Funder, R. D. Parke, C. Tomlinson-Keasey, & K. Widaman (Eds.), *Studying lives through time: Personality and development.* Washington, DC: American Psychological Association.

Sroufe, L. A., Cooper, R., & DeHart, G. (1996). *Child development: Its nature and course* (3rd ed.). New York: McGraw-Hill.

Sroufe, L. A., Schork, W., Motti, F., Lawroski, N., & Lafreniere, P. (1984). The role of affect in social competence. In C. Izard, J. Kagan, & R. Zajonc (Eds.), *Emotion, cognition, and behavior.* New York: Plenum.

Staub, E. (1971). The use of role-playing and induction in children's learning of helping and sharing behavior. *Child Development, 42,* 805–817.

Sternberg, R. J. (1984). Mechanisms of cognitive development: A componential approach. In R. J. Sternberg (Ed.), *Mechanisms of cognitive development.* New York: Freeman.

Sternberg, R. J. (1987). Teaching intelligence: The application of cognitive psychology to the improvement of intellectual skills. In J. B. Baron & R. J. Sternberg (Eds.), *Teaching thinking skills: Theory and practice.* New York: Freeman.

Stipek, D. (1993). *Motivation to learn: From theory to practice* (2nd ed.). Boston: Allyn & Bacon.

Stipek, D. (1996). Motivation and instruction. In D. Berliner & R. Calfee (Eds.), *Handbook of educational psychology.* New York: Macmillan.

Stipek, D. (1998). *Motivation to learn: From theory to practice* (3rd ed.). Boston: Allyn & Bacon.

Stipek, D., Recchia, S., & McClintic, S. (1992). Self-evaluation in young children. *Monographs of the Society for Research in Child Development, 57*(Serial No. 226).

Strayer, F. F. (1989). Co-adaptation within the early peer group: A psychobiological study of competence. In B. Schneider, G. Attili, J. Nadel, & R. Weissberg (Eds.), *Social competence in developmental perspective.* Boston: Klewer.

Strayer, F. F., Wareing, S., & Rushton, J. P. (1979). Social constraints on naturally occurring preschool altruism. *Ethology and Sociobiology, 1,* 3–11.

Stuss, D. T. (1992). Biological and psychological development of executive functions. *Brain and Cognition, 20,* 8–23.

Stuss, D., & Benson, F. (1986). *The frontal lobes.* New York: Raven.

Super, C. M., Kagan, J., Morrison, P., Haith, M., & Werffenback, J. (1972). Discrepancy and attention in the 5-month infant. *Developmental Psychology, 8,* 305-331.

Susman-Stillman, A., Kalkose, M., Egeland, B., & Waldman, I. (1996). Infant temperament and maternal sensitivity as predictors of attachment security. *Infant Behavior and Development, 19,* 13–47.

Swann, W. B. (1983). Self-verification: Bringing social reality into harmony with self. In J. Suls & A. Greenwald (Eds.), *Psychological perspectives on the self* (Vol. 2). Hillsdale, NJ: Erlbaum.

Swann, W. B. (1985). The self as architect of reality. In B. R. Schlenker (Ed.), *The self in social life.* New York: McGraw-Hill.

Swann, W. B., & Pittman, T. S. (1977). Initiating play activity of children: The moderating influence of verbal cues on intrinsic motivation. *Child Development, 48,* 1128–1132.

Sylwester, R. (1995). *A celebration of neurons: An educator's guide to the human brain.* Alexandria, VA: Association for Supervision and Curriculum Development.

Tarabulsy, G. M., Tessier, R., & Kappas, A. (1996). Contingency detection and the contingent organization of behavior in interactions: Implications for socioemotional development in infancy. *Psychological Bulletin, 120,* 25–41.

Tesser, A. (1988). Toward a self-evaluation maintenance model of social behavior. In L. Berkowitz (Ed.), *Advances in experimental social psychology* (Vol. 21). New York: Academic Press.

Thomas, A., & Chess, S. (1977). *Temperament and development.* New York: Brunner/Mazel.

Thompson, R. A. (1990). Emotion and self-regulation. In R. A. Thompson

(Ed.), *Nebraska Symposium on Motivation* (Vol. 36). Lincoln: University of Nebraska Press.

Thorndike, E. L. (1898). Animal intelligence: An experimental study of associative processes in animals. *Psychological Review Monograph Supplement, 2*(8).

Thorndike, E. L. (1911). *Animal intelligence.* New York: Macmillan.

Tomasello, M. (1996). Piagetian and Vygotskian approaches to language acquisition. *Human Development, 39,* 269–276.

Underwood, B., & Moore, B. (1982). Perspective-taking and altruism. *Psychological Bulletin, 91,* 143–173.

Urban, J., Carlson, E., Egeland, B., & Sroufe, L. A. (1991). Patterns of individual adaptation across childhood. *Development and Psychopathology, 3,* 445–460.

Valsiner, J., (Ed.) (1988). *Child development within culturally structured environments* (Vols. 1 and 2). Norwood, NJ: Ablex.

Vygotsky, L. (1962). *Thought and language.* Cambridge, MA: MIT Press.

Vygotsky, L. (1978). *Mind in society: The development of higher psychological processes.* Cambridge, MA: Harvard University Press.

Walsh, M. C., Pennington, B. F., & Grossier, D. B. (1991). A normative–developmental study of executive function: A window on prefrontal function in children. *Developmental Neuropsychology, 7,* 131–149.

Waters, E., Kondo-Ikemura, K., & Richters, J. (1990). Learning to love: Milestones and mechanisms in attachment, identity and identification. In M. Gunnar & L. A. Sroufe (Eds.), *Minnesota Symposia in Child Psychology: Vol. 23. Self processes in development.* Hillsdale, NJ: Erlbaum.

Waters, E., Wippman, J., & Sroufe, L. A. (1979). Attachment, positive affect, and competence in the peer group: Two studies in construct validation. *Child Development, 50,* 821–829).

Watson, J. S. (1966). The development and generalization of "contingency awareness" in early infancy: Some hypotheses. *Merrill-Palmer Quarterly, 12,* 123–135.

Weiner, B. (1979). A theory of motivation for some classroom experiences. *Journal of Educational Psychology, 71,* 3–25.

Weiner, B. (1985). An attributional theory of achievement motivation and emotion. *Psychological Review, 92,* 548–573.

Weiner, B. (1986). *An attributional theory of motivation and emotion.* New York: Springer-Verlag.

Wellman, H. M. (1985). The origins of metacognition. In D. Forest-Pressley, G. MacKinnon, & T. Waller (Eds.), *Metacognition, cognition, and human performance.* New York: Academic Press.

Wellman, H. M., & Estes, D. (1986). Early understanding of mental entities:

A reexamination of childhood realism. *Child Development, 57,* 910–923.

Wellman, H. M., Fabricius, W., & Sophian, C. (1985). The early development of planning. In H. Wellman (Ed.), *Children's searching: The development of search skill.* Hillsdale, NJ: Erlbaum.

Welsh, M. C., Pennington, B. F., & Groisser, D. B. (1991). A normative–developmental study of executive function: A window on prefrontal function in children. *Developmental Neuropsychology, 7,* 131–149.

Werch, J. V. (1985). *Vygotsky and the social formation of mind.* Cambridge, MA: Harvard University Press.

White, B. L. (1972). *Human infants: Experience and psychological development.* Englewood Cliffs, NJ: Prentice-Hall.

White, R. W. (1959). Motivation reconsidered: The concept of competence. *Psychological Bulletin, 104,* 36–52.

White, R. W. (1960). Competence and the psychosexual stages of development. In M. R. Jones (Ed.), *Nebraska Symposium on Motivation* (Vol. 8). Lincoln: University of Nebraska Press.

White, R. W. (1963). Ego and reality in psychoanalytic theory. *Psychological Issues, 3,* No. 3 (Monograph #11).

White, S. H. (1970). Some general outlines of the matrix of developmental changes between five and seven years. *Bulletin of the Orton Society, 20,* 41–57.

Whiting, B. B., & Edwards, C. P. (1988). *Children of different worlds: The formation of social behavior.* Cambridge, MA: Harvard University Press.

Whiting, B. B., & Whiting, J. W. M. (1975). *Children of six cultures: A psycho-cultural analysis.* Cambridge, MA: Harvard University Press.

Williams, D., & Mateer, C. A. (1992). Developmental impact of frontal lobe injury in middle childhood. *Brain and Cognition, 20,* 196–204.

Wilson, E. O. (1975). *Sociobiology.* Cambridge, MA: Harvard University Press, Belknap Press.

Wood, D., Bruner, J. S., & Ross, G. (1976). The role of tutoring in problem-solving. *Journal of Child Psychology and Psychiatry, 17,* 89–100.

Zahn-Waxler, C., & Radke-Yarrow, M. (1982). The development of altruism: Alternative strategies. In N. Eisenberg (Ed.), *The development of prosocial behavior.* New York: Academic Press.

Zahn-Waxler, C., Radke-Yarrow, M., & King, R. A. (1979). Child rearing and children's prosocial initiations toward victims of distress. *Child Development, 50,* 319–330.

Zahn-Waxler, C., Radke-Yarrow, M., Wagner, E., & Chapman, M. (1992). Development of concern for others. *Developmental Psychology, 28,* 126–136.

Zelazo, P. R., Resnick, J. S., & Pinon, D. E. (1995). Response control and the execution of verbal rules. *Developmental Psychology, 31,* 508–517.

Zimmerman, B. J. (1985). The development of "intrinsic" motivation: A social learning analysis. In G. J. Whitehurst (Ed.), *Annals of child development.* Greenwich, CT: JAI Press.

Zimmerman, B. J. (1986). Development of self-regulated learning and academic development: Which are the key subprocesses? *Contemporary Educational Psychology, 16,* 307–313.

Zimmerman, B. J. (1989). Models of self-regulated learning and academic achievement. In B. J. Zimmerman & D. H. Schunk (Eds.), *Self-regulated learning and academic achievement: Theory, research, and practice.* New York: Springer-Verlag.

Zimmerman, B. J. (1995). Self-efficacy and educational development. In A. Bandura (Ed.), *Self-efficacy in changing societies.* New York: Cambridge University Press.

Zimmerman, B. J., Bonner, S., & Kovach, R. (1996). *Developing self-regulated learners: Beyond achievement to self-efficacy.* Washington, DC: American Psychological Association.

Zimmerman, B. J., & Schunk, D. (Eds.). (1989). *Self-regulated learning and academic achievement: Theory, research, and practice.* New York: Springer-Verlag.

Zivin, G. (Ed.). (1979). *The development of self-regulation through private speech.* New York: Wiley.

Index

287